The Nail in Differential Diagnosis

The Nail in Differential Diagnosis

Robert Baran MD
Nail Disease Centre, Cannes, France

Eckart Haneke MD
Dermatology Clinic, Freiburg, Germany

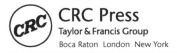

CRC Press
Taylor & Francis Group
Boca Raton London New York

CRC Press is an imprint of the
Taylor & Francis Group, an **informa** business

Traduction autorisée de l'ouvrage publié en langue anglaise sous le titre :
The Nail in Differential Diagnosis

CRC Press
Taylor & Francis Group
6000 Broken Sound Parkway NW, Suite 300
Boca Raton, FL 33487-2742

First issued in paperback 2019

© 2007 by Taylor & Francis Group, LLC
CRC Press is an imprint of Taylor & Francis Group, an Informa business

No claim to original U.S. Government works

ISBN-13: 978-1-84184-506-7 (hbk)
ISBN-13: 978-0-367-38974-1 (pbk)

Visit the Taylor & Francis Web site at
http://www.taylorandfrancis.com

and the CRC Press Web site at
http://www.crcpress.com

Contents

The nail is one of the smallest of structures, but its embryological origin and its intimate relationship with the skin render it vulnerable to disease. Its prominent position and high visibility provide a window through which we may see aspects of both local and general pathology. Its usefulness as a tool and, perhaps above all, its cosmetic features render it of utmost concern to any patient afflicted with nail disease.

It is not easy to encapsulate the differential diagnosis of nail pathology in a small book, divided somewhat artificially into ten chapters. We have attempted this daunting task by using psoriasis as a model of reference. Psoriasis may affect any or all the components of the nail apparatus. By using this disease as our framework and by discussing its pathological effect on the nail, we have attempted to broaden the field to the general pathological picture of nail disease and its differential diagnosis.

Taking advantage of the universal effect of psoriasis in this region, we have endeavoured to elaborate on the pathology of each component of the nail apparatus and its susceptibility to the wide variety of diseases that may be manifest in this intriguing organ.

We thank the many friends who have helped us in this task for the excellent illustrations which, we hope, will clarify the text beyond the capacity of the written word.

Robert Baran
Eckart Haneke

Chapter 1

Pits, rough nails, and other surface alterations

Psoriasis is the dermatosis that most frequently affects the nail. At any time, approximately 30–50% of all psoriatic subjects have nail alterations,[1] and over the course of their life, about 90% of all psoriatics will develop psoriatic nail changes. Psoriasis can affect virtually all nail structures, both singly and in combination. Thus, a considerable number of different modifications are possible. Taking into account that almost every psoriatic has 'his or her own form of psoriasis', there are so many clinical possibilities that the psoriatic lesions can mimic or at least resemble a great number of other ungual lesions due to other diseases, tumors, and trauma. Hence, it follows that psoriasis is an excellent model to show the spectrum of nail lesions and their differential diagnosis.

Pits and striations are the most common surface alterations of the nail plate (Figure 1.1). The anatomy and biology of the nail indicate that these must arise from a change to the most proximal, or so-called dorsal, matrix. Short-lived alterations will lead to round or oval lesions, and longstanding alterations to longitudinal lesions. Larger pits with smooth margins are called **depressions**, while even larger ones due to wearing down, are called **surface depressions** (Figure 1.2), or 'usure des ongles'. Horizontal splits develop when interlammellar bridges separate. The existence of a large number of small surface depressions leads to rough-surfaced nails – these may be a sign of psoriasis, alopecia areata, lichen planus, eczema, atopic dermatitis, or immunoglobulin A (IgA) deficiency.[2] Transverse grooves, first described in 1797 by Reil after high fever and described again in 1848 by Beau,[3] are due to a transitory slowdown in the rate of nail formation. A temporary

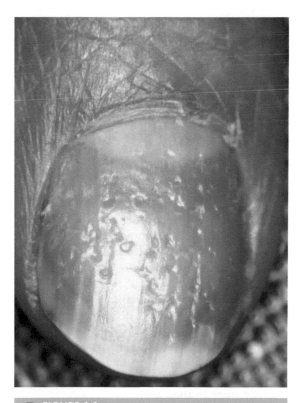

Common nail pitting.

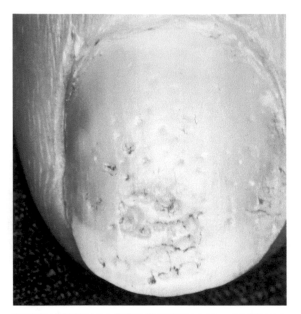

■ FIGURE 1.2

Nail depressions.

complete halt to nail formation (Figure 1.3) will lead to a defect of the nail plate called **ony-chomadesis**. Deep longitudinal defects due to a lack of continuity of the nail plate are called **splits** or **fissures**.

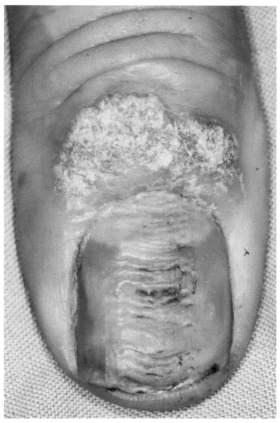

■ FIGURE 1.3

Transverse grooves. (Courtesy of B Richert, Belgium.)

■■■ DERMATOSES

Psoriasis is one of the most common geneti-cally determined immune-mediated skin diseases, affecting roughly 2% of the world population. The clinical appearance is typical in most cases, both for lesions of glabrous and palmoplantar skin and for scalp and nails. Except for the semi-mucosa of the glans penis, mucous membranes are usually spared. Nail involvement is common. About 50% of psoriasis patients consulting a der-matologist present with ungual alterations, and 90% of all psoriatics will develop nail lesions at least once in their life.

Pits (foveolae psoriaticae) are the com-monest and most reliable signs of **nail psoria-sis** (Table 1.1). Pits of relatively equal size, about 1–1.5 mm in diameter, and round (like the impression of a small round ball) are typical of nail psoriasis. They may occur singly or in large numbers almost covering the whole nail (Figures 1.4 and 1.5). Although pits may occur in many different conditions (and also without any known disease) the presence of 20 or more pits is indicative of psoriasis.[4] These pits are usually arranged in an apparently random fashion, but they may occur in transverse rows resembling Beau–Reil lines (Figure 1.6). These rows of pits may be irregular (Figure 1.7), but may also rarely be arranged in a regular pattern resembling a checkerboard. However, it is not uncommon to

Importance of pits and onycholysis for the diagnostis of psoriasis[9]

- A psoriatic origin for nail dystrophy is indicated by at least two of the following: nail pitting, horizontal ridging, and onycholysis
- The presence or absence of nail pitting alone is a poor discriminator between psoriatic and other causes of nail dystrophy
- More than 20 fingernail pits per person is suggestive of a psoriatic cause of nail dystrophy
- More than 60 pits per person are unlikely to be found in the absence of psoriasis
- Onycholysis alone in the absence of previous disease of the distal nail bed or injury to the affected nail favors a psoriatic origin for the nail dystrophy if manicure-induced onycholysis semilunaris can be excluded

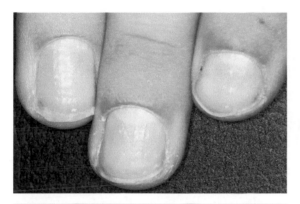

■ FIGURE 1.4

Psoriatic pitting involving several nails.

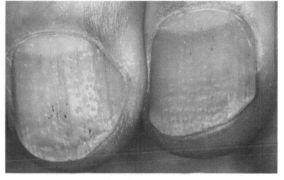

■ FIGURE 1.6

Vertical pitting on a left psoriatic nail and horizontal pitting on the right nail.

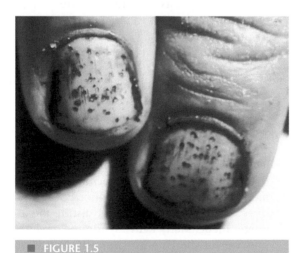

■ FIGURE 1.5

Psoriatic pitting after anthralin treatment, which makes the pits more visible.

see some pits arranged in a longitudinal fashion, commonly in a single row.

Psoriatic pits develop from tiny psoriatic lesions located in the most proximal portion of the matrix, which is responsible for the formation of the dorsal nail plate. The psoriatic lesion causes a tiny area of parakeratosis on the surface of the newly formed nail, which can be easily seen on histological slides. When, during nail growth, this parakeratosis emerges from under the proximal nail fold, it breaks out from the normal orthokeratotic nail plate, leaving a tiny pit in the plate. This mechanism of formation explains why the pit is not a true depression, but rather a defect of nail plate substance – hence the term 'psoriatic erosion'. The intensity of the psoriatic process and its transverse extension determine the depth and transverse diameter of the

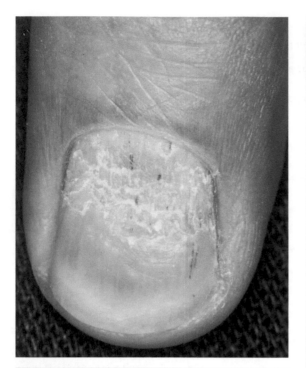

■ FIGURE 1.7

Irregular pitting and depression in a psoriatic nail.

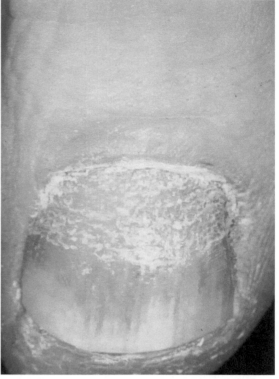

■ FIGURE 1.8

Pits emerging from beneath the proximal nail fold and retaining parakeratotic cells.

pit, whereas its duration and severity determine the longitudinal diameter. Sometimes, the parakeratosis remains in the pits for several weeks (Figures 1.8 and 1.9).

Often, some pits are arranged in a longitudinal manner indicating that there might be a repeated irritation to a particular small area of the matrix, whereas pits arranged in a transverse manner resembling Reil–Beau lines may be due to a more general stimulus.

Depressions of the nail plate surface similar to those seen in psoriasis are quite common. A single pit either smaller, of the same size, or larger than a typical psoriatic pit may occur spontaneously without association with any other disease. However, when pits occur on several fingers and repeatedly, psoriasis should be suspected even without a positive family and/or personal history of psoriasis. The histogenesis of these incidental pits is not yet known.

Single deep pits are also sometimes seen in onychomycosis, but to a much lesser degree than in psoriasis. They may occasionally be seen in candidal and other types of paronychia (see below and Chapter 5).

A few pits, with an irregular distribution, are seen during infectious diseases and are sometimes called **Rosenau's sign**.

Reiter syndrome is characterized by the classical triad of ocular, genital, and oral mucosal lesions with rheumatoid arthritis-like joint lesions, which may be incapacitating. It was formerly divided into a post-gonorrhoeal and an intestinal type; however, this distinction is no longer made. Many Reiter syndrome patients are positive for the HLA-B27 antigen. Nail changes in Reiter syndrome may mimic ungual psoriasis for a long time (Figure 1.10). These usually start

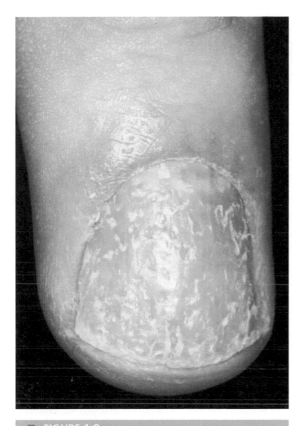

■ FIGURE 1.9

Diffuse pitting with parakeratotic cells.

with pits and salmon spots. The latter, however, are often more brownish than in classical psoriasis, due to the presence of more extravasated erythrocytes.[5] An aspect like paronychia may be the first sign of nail involvement (Figure 1.11).

A case of a father and his 6-year-old son who were both positive for HLA-A2 and B27 was described in which the father had Reiter syndrome with chronic arthritis, recurrent anterior uveitis, amyloidosis, and a transplanted kidney, whereas the boy had only nail changes suggestive of Reiter syndrome; no psoriasis-associated antigens were found.[6]

Pits (trachyonychia) are a characteristic feature of **nail eczema** (Figures 1.12 and 1.13) that is independent of the type of eczema – although pits are more common in allergic contact and nummular eczema than in atopic dermatitis.[7] They are usually less well circumscribed and shallower, and they may occur in large numbers sufficient to cause a roughening of the nail surface. Depressions are larger and have a less well delimited margin than pits. Quite often, they do not lose their shine, even in the depth of the depression. Subungual allergic contact dermatitis, in contrast, does not cause pitting, but rather subungual hyperkeratosis and onycholysis.[8]

Shiny fingernails (unguis lucidus) (Figure 1.14) are typical of patients with atopic eczema and other chronic itching dermatoses: a

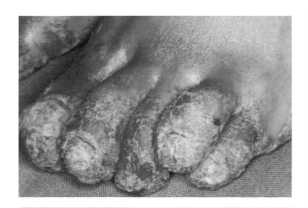

■ FIGURE 1.10

Reiter syndrome.

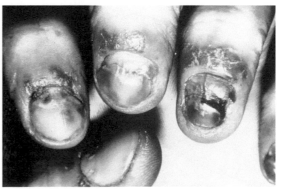

■ FIGURE 1.11

Reiter syndrome with paronychia.

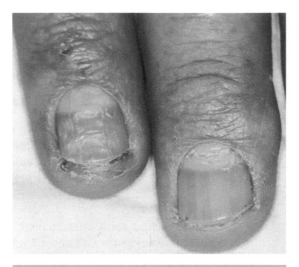

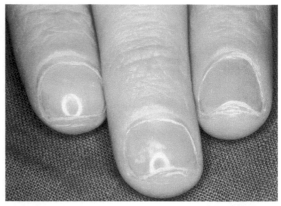

Shiny finger nails associated with itching chronic dermatitis. (Courtesy of B Schubert, France.)

Irregular pits in contact dermatitis.

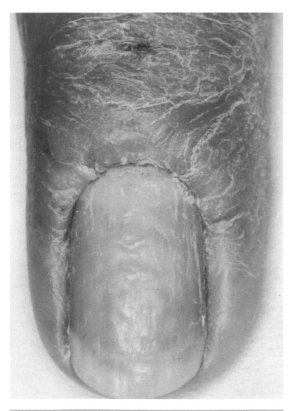

Contact dermatitis.

patient rubs the itchy skin with the dorsa of the distal phalanges and thus polishes the nails. This is even more pronounced when greasy skin is rubbed or particularly when soft oily zinc paste preparations are applied before rubbing.

The nail plate is remarkably permeable to water. It can swell very rapidly and takes up more water than the stratum corneum of the epidermis. Transonychial water loss by evaporation is therefore a constant feature. Peculiarly, transonychial water loss has been found to be reduced in nail eczema, psoriasis, and onychomycosis; this is thought to be due to the formation of a granular layer in the diseased matrix and nail bed, in contrast to epidermis, where inflammation usually induces parakeratosis and increases transepidermal water loss.

Alopecia areata is a relatively common autoimmune disorder with characteristic round bald spots. Although the scalp is most frequently involved, any part of the hairy skin may be affected. Nail involvement in alopecia areata is quite common: occurring in over 10% of adults and over 25% of children. It is said that the more severe the alopecia, the more likely is nail involvement, and this is of considerable prognostic significance.[9,10] Thus, nail involvement is seen much more frequently in alopecia universalis than in circumscribed alopecia areata.

However, exclusive ungual alopecia areata probably does exist. The linear nail growth is slower than in psoriasis. The nail surface is covered by small pits and longitudinal striations, and the plate is often slightly thickened, grayish, no longer transparent, and brittle (Figures 1.15–1.17). The rough surface may keep its luster, but in the majority of cases, the nail shine is lost.

Both nail eczema and ungual alopecia areata are histologically spongiotic dermatitis of the matrix (and nail bed) with exudation of serum, which becomes incorporated into the nail plate. Spongiotic vesicles typical of contact dermatitis also form in the nail matrix and nail bed. When they are localized in the proximal matrix, they

will dry when growing out with the nail and leave a depression in the nail plate surface. When the spongiosis is more prominent in the central and distal parts of the matrix, the serous exudates become incorporated into the nail plate, giving rise to nail thickening, brittleness, loss of transparency, and a grayish colour. Probably even more important for the roughened appearance of the nail is the fact that the inflammation and incorporation of serum and inflammatory cells cause a wavy arrangement of the onychocytes and their keratin fibers, in contrast to the regular linear arrangement in normal nail plates.

Causes of nail pitting (trachyonychia) are summarized in Table 1.2.

The hallmark of **20-nail dystrophy** is trachyonychia of (almost) all nails; however, it is

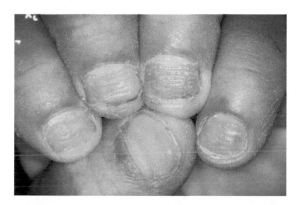

■ FIGURE 1.15

Horizontal pitting in alopecia areata.

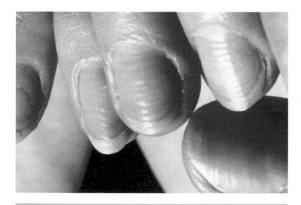

■ FIGURE 1.16

Tranverse lines in alopecia areata.

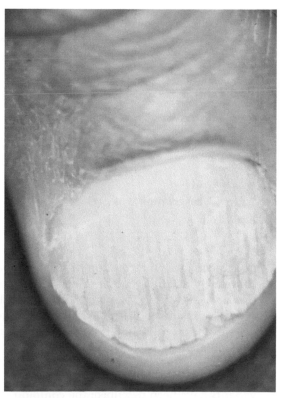

■ FIGURE 1.17

Rough surface in alopecia areata.

■ TABLE 1.2

Causes of nail pitting

Causes	Features
Most common	
Psoriasis vulgaris	Regular, few to innumerable, sometimes arranged in lines
Alopecia areata	Shallow; if present in great number, may cause trachyonychia
Eczema	Irregular in size and arrangement
Occupational injury	Irregular, few
Reiter syndrome	Similar to psoriasis
Onychomycosis	Few, irregular in size and distribution
Less common	
Acute rheumatic fever	
Chronic mucocutaneous candidosis	Few to extremely abundant, all sizes, worm-eaten aspect
Diabetes mellitus	
Infectious diseases in general; dermatophytosis	
Lichen nitidus	Rare
Lichen planus	Very fine, often causing aspect of longitudinal ridging
Normal nail	Very few, irregular in size and distribution
Paronychia	
Pemphigus foliaceus	
Pemphigus vulgaris	
Peripheral vascular disease	Rare
Pityriasis rosea	Few, irregular
Sarcoidosis	Rare
Secondary syphilis	
Systemic lupus erythematosus (SLE)	
Tuberculosis (active)	

not uncommon that one or two nails remain completely unaffected over a period of sometimes several years. The nature of this peculiar condition is not yet clear.[11] While some authors defend this term because it denotes a condition with different possible etiologies, others recommend discarding it because it includes a wide variety of different disorders.[12] Three clinical variants have been described: the common variant with densely situated pits, a 'sandpapered' nail with a lusterless rough surface caused by excessive longitudinal ridging as if the nail surface had been rubbed vertically with coarse sandpaper, and a shiny variant with pits.[13] In most cases, histopathology shows a spongiotic dermatitis.[14] Twenty-nail dystrophy is not discernable from widespread involvement of alopecia areata (Figure 1.18), either clinically or histologically, although histopathology may reveal or exclude another cause such as lichen planus.[15] Jerasutus et al[16] consider it to be a specific localization of atopic dermatitis in the nail matrix.

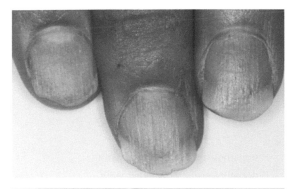

■ **FIGURE 1.18**

Trachyonychia in alopecia areata 20-nail dystrophy.

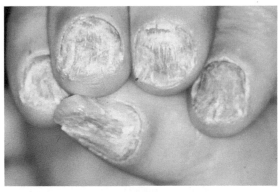

■ **FIGURE 1.19**

Trachyonychia in psoriatic 20-nail dystrophy.

Similar clinical features may also be shown by psoriasis (Figure 1.19) and nail lichen planus[17] (Figure 1.20). Koilonychia may develop in the course of 20-nail dystrophy. Whether or not associated conditions such as vitiligo, incontinentia pigmenti, ichthyosis vulgaris, knuckle pads, chromosomal translocation, IgA deficiency, or other autoimmune disorders have a causal relationship with 20-nail dystrophy or are just chance associations is not yet clear. Twenty-nail dystrophy has also been observed in monozygotic twins, and familial as well as hereditary cases have been described. The etiology and associations of trachyonychia are summarized in Table 1.3.

Ridging of the nail plate surface is also seen in psoriasis, although much less frequently than pitting. On the other hand, ridging and grooving are typical signs of aging, often beginning as early as during the fourth decade. Small beads of keratin may develop in a longitudinal arrangement, reflecting a permanent though alternating disturbance of keratinization in the proximal matrix.[18] Histologically, the ridges overlie the elevated ridges of the nail bed and the beads correspond to round pertinax bodies characterized by whirled keratin. In extreme old age, the nail surface also loses its shine, and the fingernail plate gradually becomes thinner and fragile, with parallel longitudinal fissures.

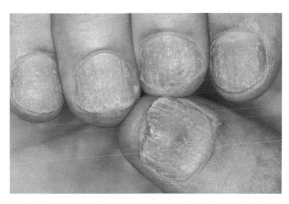

■ **FIGURE 1.20**

Trachyonychia in lichen planus 20-nail dystrophy.

Nail involvement is relatively common in **lichen planus**, although this latter condition may also be limited to the nail plates[19] or associated with oral mucosa[20], as has been documented by histological studies.[21] The nail involvement may be the initial and most important clinical manifestation of the disease process, and permanent anonychia (complete loss of the nail) may result. Longitudinal ridging is most typical of lichen planus, where the involved nail plate may look as if the surface had been treated vigorously with coarse sandpaper[22–25] (Figure 1.21). Fine, densely arranged (Figure 1.22) longitudinal grooves and ridges give this rough surface appearance. The nail plate loses its shine and may

■ **TABLE 1.3**

Etiology and associations of trachyonychia

Causes	Features
Alopecia areata	Histopathology: spongiotic dermatitis
Amyloidosis	Histopathology: amyloidosis
Chromosomal translocation	
Ectodermal dysplasia	
Eczema, atopic dermatitis	Histopathology: spongiotic dermatitis
Graft-versus-host disease	Histopathology: interface dermatitis
Hematological abnormalities	
Ichthyosis vulgaris	
Incontinentia pigmenti	
Lichen planus	Histopathology: interface dermatitis
Psoriasis	Histopathology: psoriasis
Red lunulae and knuckle pads	
Selective immunoglobulin A deficiency	
Vitiligo	Autoimmune process ?
Hereditary: monozygotic twins; familial cases	Autosomal dominant ?

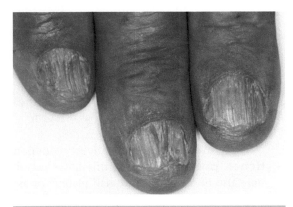

■ **FIGURE 1.21**

Longitudinal ridging with nail splitting in lichen planus.

become opaque. Lichen planus-like cutaneous side-effects of β-blockers and other drugs including captopril and other angiotensin-converting enzyme (ACE) inhibitors, brimonide collyrium, and mercury amalgam may involve the nail. Histologically, lichen planus of the nail is characterized by a dense band-like epidermotropic infiltrate of the proximal matrix and adjacent

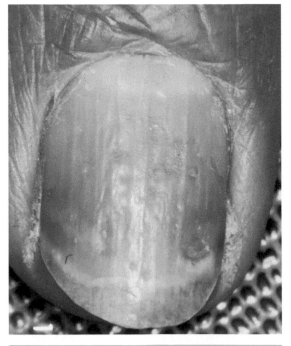

■ **FIGURE 1.22**

Irregular pitting in lichen planus.

epithelium of the undersurface of the proximal nail fold. The basal cell layer shows a hydropic degeneration typical of lichen planus, which leads insidiously to epithelial thinning and decreased nail formation. Since the dorsal layer of the nail plate is responsible for the nail shine, it is self-evident that the involvement of the most proximal matrix portion causes a loss of luster. This process is irreversible, and leads eventually to cicatricial obliteration of the nail cul-de-sac and to nail atrophy. It may even progress to anonychia.[26]

Causes of anonychia are summarized in Table 1.4.

When the hydropic basal cell degeneration is very pronounced, bullous lichen planus of the nails may exceptionally result. The nail surface is rough, but the nail plate is thickened, overcurved, and yellow.[27]

Nail involvement appears to be rare in childhood lichen planus.

Graft-versus-host disease (GVHD) may exhibit a clinical and histological pattern of nail changes that is very similar to that of lichen planus (Figures 1.23 and 1.24). When affected, the nails become dull, lose their shine, and develop longitudinal striations and ridging. Acute onset of the disease also causes Reil–Beau lines. However, with time, and particularly dur-

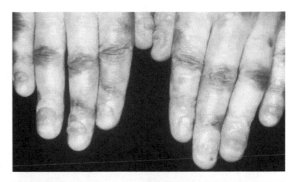

■ FIGURE 1.23

Chronic graft-versus-host disease. (Courtesy of O Correia, Portugal.)

ing and after therapy, the inflammatory infiltrate will almost disappear and give way to an almost acellular reaction. Differential diagnostic problems with dyskeratosis congenita may arise when there is also a reticulate pigmentation of the skin.

Amyloidosis, both primary and associated with plasmocytoma, can affect the nail. Nail changes may even be the first sign of amyloidosis[28,29] (Figures 1.25 and 1.26). Typically, the nail is thin and brittle, with longitudinal ridges and distal splits. Narrow, pink longitudinal subungual striations and splinter hemorrhages as well as subungual hematomas may occur. Nail loss has

---

■ TABLE 1.4

Causes of anonychia

Hereditary	Acquired
May be autosomal dominant or autosomal recessive	Diphenylhydantoin
	Allergic reaction to acrylic nail preparations
Anonychia and ectrodactyly (autosomal dominant)	Teratogens during pregnancy cause anonychia
Coffin–Siris syndrome (anonychia, ectrodactyly, mental retardation)	at birth: alcohol, phenytoin
Focal dermal hypoplasia	
Darier's disease	
Nail–patella syndrome	
Congenital onychodysplasia of the index fingers	

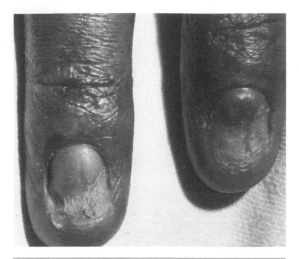

■ FIGURE 1.24

Lichen planus-like ulcerative changes (graft-versus-host disease). (Courtesy of JH Saurat, Switzerland.)

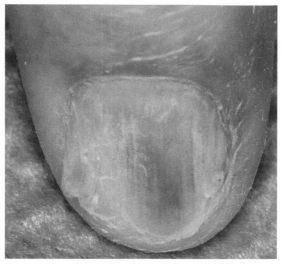

■ FIGURE 1.26

Erythronychia in amyloidosis. (Courtesy of C Cholez, France.)

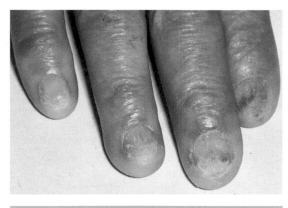

■ FIGURE 1.25

Lichen planus-like nail changes in amyloidosis.

been observed. Rarely, the nails are thickened and shiny. Nail biopsy reveals typical amyloid deposits, which are conspicuous by their yellowish-green birefringence under polarized light.[30]

A case of autosomal dominant nail changes with marked thickening and yellow discoloration associated with macular cutaneous amyloidosis has been described. The nail alterations resolved during the third and fourth decades of life.

Lichen striatus (Figure 1.27) may involve the whole nail or just a portion. Longitudinal striation identical to that in lichen planus is typical. In the case of complete nail involvement, differentiation from lichen planus may be impossible.[31] Nail involvement is often associated with a more protracted course of the lesions of lichen striatus, and therefore differential diagnosis with ILVEN (Inflammatory Linear Verrucous Epidermal Nevus) may be difficult, and the latter may even be considered as a variant of lichen striatus.[32]

The nails in **scleroderma** often exhibit loss of shine and some ridging, particularly in acrosclerosis and the CREST (Calcinosis, Raynaud's phenomenon, Esophageal involvement, Sclerodactyly, Telangiectasia) syndrome. **Lupus erythematosus** may also exhibit loss of shine and fine longitudinal striations.

Causes of longitudinal ridging are summarized in Table 1.5.

Squamous cell carcinoma in situ (Bowen's disease and epidermoid carcinoma) may involve the matrix and cause disturbed nail plate formation with roughness and longitudinal

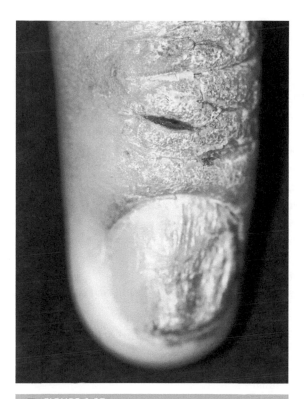

■ FIGURE 1.27

Lichen striatus. (Courtesy of R Arenas, Mexico DF.)

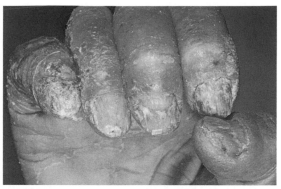

■ FIGURE 1.28

Acrokeratosis paraneoplastica: psoriasis-like changes.

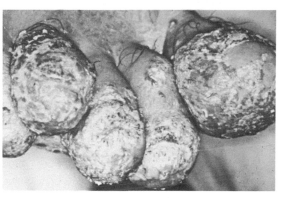

■ FIGURE 1.29

Acrokeratosis paraneoplastica: psoriasis-like changes.

striation, usually on one side of a nail only.[33] Leukonychia has also been observed in Bowen's disease.

Nail dystrophy is a typical sign of **acrokeratosis paraneoplastica of Bazex–Dupré**[34,35] (Figures 1.28 and 1.29). This paraneoplastic syndrome is characterized by slowly evolving psoriasiform erythematous to violaceous lesions of the nose, the external ear, the hands, the feet, and the periungual skin. The nails may become striated, opaque, and brittle, sometimes with distal subungual hyperkeratosis. Rarely, vesicles, bullae, and crusts develop. The condition is associated with malignancies of the upper aerodigestive tract, and in almost two-thirds of cases precedes the detection of the cancer by 10–12 months; thus, early recognition of this characteristic paraneoplastic syndrome would allow much earlier diagnosis of the underlying neoplasm. Cachexia often develops before the correct diagnosis is made. More than 90% of patients are male, with an average age of 60 years. The skin and nail lesions are resistant to topical treatment, but the cutaneous alterations usually disappear with tumor removal and reappear with cancer recurrence, whereas the nail lesions do not regress. The pathogenesis remains enigmatic. An autoimmune process has been suggested.

Chronic mucocutaneous candidosis is a group of rare immune defects characterized by early-onset infection with *Candida albicans*, usually postnatally or in infancy, and running an extremely protracted course. From early infancy, scalp, glabrous skin, oral and genital mucosa,

■ TABLE 1.5

Causes of longitudinal ridging

Causes	Features
Age	Very frequent, often insidiously exhibiting beading also (pertinax bodies)
Trauma	Usually only one or a few lines
Median canaliform dystrophy	Central longitudinal break with proximally directed oblique lines originating from this central line
Lichen planus	Fine dense longitudinal ridging with loss of nail shine
Lichen striatus	Usually only one finger affected, often only partially
Graft-versus-host disease	Dense longitudinal ridging
Amyloidosis	Dense longitudinal ridging
Mycosis fungoides, Sézary syndrome	Dull brittle nails with longitudinal striations; often also splinter hemorrhages
Psoriasis	Relatively rare; may be associated with pitting
Dyskeratosis follicularis	White and red longitudinal lines; often with a notch at the free nail plate margin
Hailey–Hailey disease	Multiple whitish lines
Scleroderma	Fine longitudinal ridges and loss of shine and transparency
Lupus erythematosus	Fine longitudinal lines
Leprosy	56% in paucibacillary, 83% in multibacillary
Nail–patella syndrome	One or several lines or fissures
Frostbite	Fine lines
X-irradiation	Loss of nail shine; fine lines developing into fissures, splinter hemorrhages
Poor arterial circulation	Loss of nail shine; fine lines
Rheumatoid arthritis	Loss of nail shine; fine lines
Onychomycosis	Irregular, sometimes with yellow color (dermatophytoma)
Tumors:	Size and number depend on tumor
Koenen tumors	One or few canaliform depressions; increase in number and width with time
Nail fibrokeratoma (FK)	Usually one wide canaliform depression when FK originates from the most proximal matrix (eponychial fibrokeratoma)
	Longitudinal depression breaks out the nail plate distal to the free margin of the proximal nail fold when the origin is in the proximal to medial part of the matrix (intraungual or dissecting FK)
	Longitudinal rim when FK originates from the most distal matrix or proximal nail bed (subungual FK)
Myxoid pseudocyst	Wide shallow longitudinal depression; may develop irregularities when the cyst ruptures
Bowen's disease	Whitish color with irregular ridging according to the involved portion of the matrix
Glomus tumor	Red longitudinal stripe with slight elevation of the nail plate

and nails may be affected. Huge, often grotesquely hyperkeratotic, lesions may develop on the scalp and extremities, and chronic hyperplastic oral candidosis with recalcitrant angular cheilitis is typical. The nail apparatus develops total dystrophic onychomycosis (Figure 1.30), often with granulomatous inflammation and pseudoclubbing (Figure 1.31); another feature of the nail involvement is a peculiar surface alteration resembling worm-eaten wood.[36] Histological examinations have shown that the matrix and nail bed are severely inflamed and only form keratotic debris instead of normal nail material. This has also been confirmed by electron microscopy.

A rough and lusterless nail surface, often with shallow transverse grooves on one or both sides of the nail, is common in **chronic paronychia** of different origins. Growth of bacteria and some yeasts may stain the lateral aspect of the nail dirty grayish to black (see below).

Onychomycosis due to dermatophytes (Figure 1.32) and some nondermatophyte molds may also cause an irregular surface with some pits, loss of shine and transparency, and brittleness.

A rough, sandpapered-like appearance of the nail may be seen in nail **lichen nitidus**.[37,38]

Pityriasis rubra pilaris usually presents with thick, gray, and striated nails; the more the skin lesions are pronounced on the dorsa of the fingers, the more severe are the nail lesions.[39,40] The hyponychium may show pronounced hyperkeratosis (Figure 1.33).

Keratotic scabies[41,42] (Figure 1.34) shows a lack of nail luster and marked thickening of the hyponychial keratin. There may be associated psoriasiform changes of the tips of the digits.

Parakeratosis pustulosa of Hjorth–Sabouraud[43,44] (Figure 1.35), which commonly occurs in young girls, starts with some pustules near the free margin of the nail. These develop into eczematoid changes of the skin with fine scaling, until a marked hyperkeratosis of the distal nail bed develops and lifts up the nail. Pitting

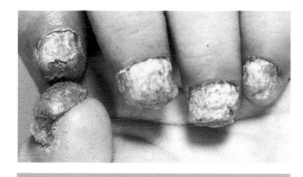

■ FIGURE 1.30

Chronic mucocutaneous candidosis. (Courtesy of CS Seow, Singapore.)

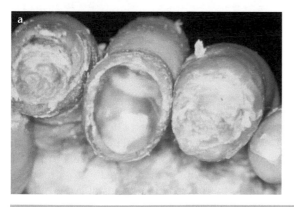
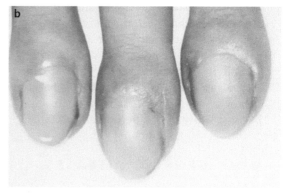

■ FIGURE 1.31

(a) Chronic mucocutaneous candidosis associated with pseudo-clubbing. (b) The same patient after treatment (itraconazole).

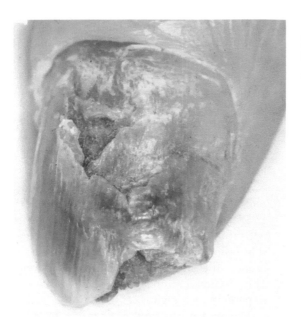

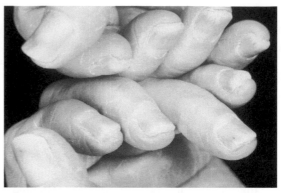

Pityriasis rubra pilaris. (Courtesy of A Griffiths, UK.)

■ FIGURE 1.32

Total dystrophic onychomycosis.

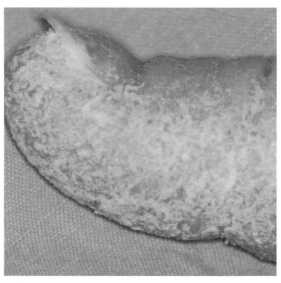

and more rarely transverse ridging occur. Histology shows both psoriasiform and eczematoid alterations: hyperkeratosis, parakeratosis, pustulation, acanthosis, papillomatosis, exocytosis, and a dense, mainly lymphocytic infiltrate around capillaries. Recently, a series of 20 patients with the clinical diagnosis of parakeratosis pustulosa was examined, and the authors concluded that this clinical diagnosis was not an entity but rather a sign of psoriasis, contact dermatitis, or atopic dermatitis.[45]

Rough nails may also be observed in **Brazilian pemphigus (fogo selvagem)**; however, with this condition, nails may also become shiny due to permanent rubbing.

■■■ **GENETIC DISEASES**

Longitudinal striation is also typical of **dyskeratosis follicularis (Darier's disease)**. In addition, white and sometimes reddish longitudinal stripes may be seen that may lead to small V-

■ FIGURE 1.34

Keratotic scabies. (Courtesy of D Van Neste, Belgium.)

shaped notches in the free margin of the nail with a tendency towards longitudinal tears and splits[46,47] (Figure 1.36). The mechanism behind this appearance is typical papule formation on the skin being transformed into grooves and ridges by the proximal to distal growth direction of the nail.

Nail involvement in **benign familial pemphigus of Hailey–Hailey** is clinically and histologically similar to that of dyskeratosis fol-

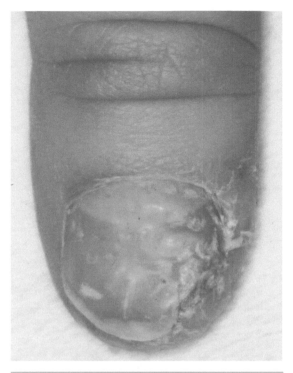

■ FIGURE 1.35
Parakeratosis pustulosa (Hjorth–Sabouraud).

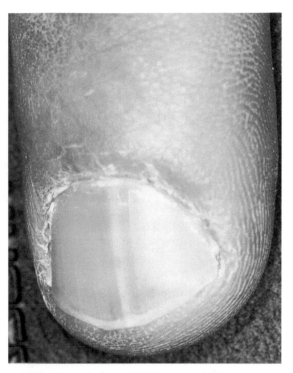

■ FIGURE 1.37
Longitudinal leukonychia in Hailey–Hailey disease.

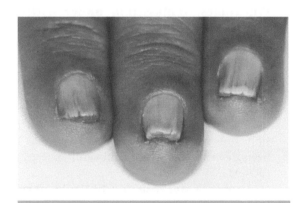

■ FIGURE 1.36
Darier's disease.

licularis, but the typical V-shaped notches of Darier's disease are not commonly seen and only the white longitudinal stripes are observed[48] (Figure 1.37).

Rough distal nails have been observed in **familial koilonychia**, with loss of luster and thin, dark nails. The brown discoloration becomes more intense with age. Parakeratotic cells have been found in the middle of the nail plate.[49]

Longitudinal ridging, onychorrhexis, onychoschizia, trachyonychia, and notching have been described in hereditary **punctate palmoplantar keratoderma of Brauer–Buschke–Fischer**[50] (Figure 1.38). Pitting, onycholysis, and subungual hyperkeratosis have been seen in another two cases.[51] An otherwise undefined nail dystrophy has been described in a patient with **epidermolysis bullosa simplex with mottled pigmentation** and peculiar punctate keratoses of the fingers.[52]

A recently described case of **keratosis follicularis spinulosa decalvans**, a disease linked to chromosome Xp22.13–22.2, showed marked

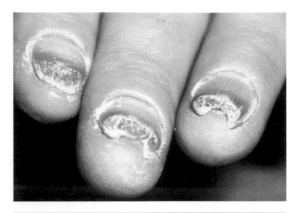

Subungual hyperkeratosis in punctate palmoplantar keratoderma.

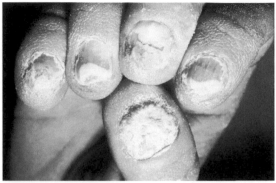

Keratosis–ichthyosis–deafness (KID) syndrome. (Courtesy of G Badillet, France.)

dystrophy of finger- and toenails, with thickening and irregular transverse lines and grooves.[53] In addition, the patient had almost generalized alopecia, focal keratoderma of the palms and soles, blepharitis, ectropium, and photophobia. The nail changes appear to be associated with 'highly placed' cuticles.[54]

Other syndromes with nail dystrophy, follicular hyperkeratosis, and ocular symptoms include the **keratosis–ichthyosis–deafness (KID)** (Figure 1.39) and **ichthyosis follicularis with atrichia and photosensitivity (IFAP) syndromes.**

Nail dystrophy is also seen in **hereditary mucoepithelial dysplasia**, which is otherwise characterized clinically by beefy red oral, nasal, and vaginal mucosa, with dyskeratosis, lack of cohesion of the epithelium, and cytoplasmic vacuoles. These mucosal changes are the cause of the frequent respiratory tract complications, including chronic rhinitis, recurrent pneumonia, pneumothorax, and terminal lung disease.[55]

Longitudinal ridging has been seen in a case of an **X-linked polyendocrinopathy–immune dysregulation syndrome**.[56]

Transverse grooving has been seen in a case of **Papillon–Lefèvre syndrome**.[57] It is also a feature of **Heimler syndrome**, which is characterized by sensorineural hearing loss, enamel hypoplasia of the teeth, Reil–Beau lines, and leukonychia.[58]

■■■ SYSTEMIC CONDITIONS

The nail changes in **Klinefelter syndrome, chronic malnutrition** and/or **vitamin A deficiency, Job syndrome, malabsorption syndromes, thalassemia under hydroxyurea treatment**, and other debilitating conditions are usually nonspecific. The nails may become rough, soft and/or brittle, lose their shine, or become ridged, and the latter two conditions particularly may cause pigmented longitudinal streaks. The nail changes described in **Cronkhite–Canada syndrome** are most possibly due to malnutrition,[59] and this has also been described in a case of juvenile polyps and cachexia.

Anorexia nervosa and **bulimia nervosa** lead to severe alimentary deficiencies, with nail changes in almost half of the patients. Hyperkeratoses on the dorsal aspect of the fingers are known as Russel's sign in bulimia and are due to the mechanical irritation of inserting the fingers into the mouth to induce vomiting.

Nail dystrophy leading to pterygium formation is seen rarely in **sarcoidosis**, and occurs mainly in association with underlying bone alterations.[60,61]

Glucagonoma (Figure 1.40) commonly leads to characteristic periorificial erosive skin lesions known as **necrolytic migratory erythema (glucagonoma syndrome)**.[62] Very similar skin lesions are also seen in zinc deficiency and early pellagra, as well as the carboxylase-resistant biotinidase deficiency syndrome. The nails become thin, folded, opaque, and extremely brittle, and show onychorrhexis.

Horizontal splits and grooves may be observed to grow out from under the nail in **hypoparathyroidism**.[63] These changes have been attributed to the hypocalcemia that occurs due to parathyroid deficiency. Hypoparathyroidism may also be associated with other endocrinopathies and mucocutaneous candidosis and causes loss of nail shine and distal longitudinal splits.

A severe generalized disease such as **high fever** will slow down the rate of nail formation and cause a transverse groove, called **Reil–Beau lines** (Figure 1.41). These are most pronounced on the rapidly growing fingernails and are seen much less frequently on the slowly growing toenails. Repeated development of these lines points to a cyclical cause.[64] In neonates, transverse grooves are often seen from week 5 on, and are most pronounced on the thumb. They move distally, reaching the free nail margins at weeks 12–15. Occurrence on only one hand points to a cause restricted to this extremity (e.g. subclavian syndrome or carpal tunnel syndrome). They are seen quite commonly on only one finger some weeks after an operation.

Longitudinal ridging and transverse striations are common in leprosy; nail changes were seen in 56% of 150 patients with paucibacillary leprosy and in 87% of 150 patients with multibacillary disease.[65]

Causes of transverse ridges and depressions are summarized in Table 1.6 and the associations of Reil–Beau lines are described in Table 1.7.

In **mycosis fungoides**, and particularly in **Sézary syndrome**, the nail may become dull, opaque, and brittle, and may develop surface alterations almost indistinguishable from trachyonychia. In addition, splinter hemorrhages may be seen.

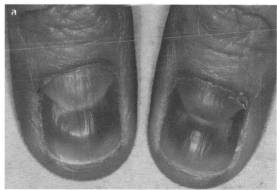

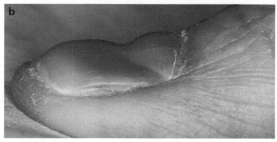

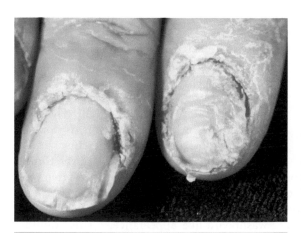

■ FIGURE 1.40

Glucagonoma. (Courtesy of J Jelinek, USA.)

■ FIGURE 1.41

(a) Beau's lines. (b) Beau's lines, same patient.

■ TABLE 1.6

Causes of transverse ridges and depressions

Disease	Type of ridges / depressions
Reil–Beau lines	Transverse depression running parallel to the lunula border
	• When all nails are involved: acute severe systemic disease, intoxication, certain deficiency states, postnatal radiotherapy (depending on dose delivered)
	• When occurring at regular intervals: menstrual cycle, chemotherapy cycles
	• When only upper extremities are involved: acute arterial occlusion
	• When only one extremity is involved: extremity tourniquet (surgery), carpal tunnel syndrome, Takayasu's disease
	• When only one digit is involved: previous surgery of the digit
Contact dermatitis, eczema	Usually irregular, mostly fingernails
Alopecia areata	Usually developing from pits that are arranged in regular lines
Psoriasis	Developing from pits that are arranged in regular lines or due to associated paronychia
Erythema multiforme	When tip of digit is involved
Stevens–Johnson syndrome	Either through systemic effect or when tip of digit is involved
Lyell syndrome	Different degrees of severity: from shallow transverse furrow, to onychomadesis, to complete temporary or even permanent loss of the nails
Congenital malalignment of the big toenail	Hallux nails exclusively involved, with oyster-shell appearance, lateral deviation, onycholysis, greenish discoloration
Trauma:	
Single	Only injured finger involved, degree depends on severity of trauma, deviation, onycholysis, greenish discoloration
Multiple	Usually irregular involvement, often only the thumb(s), with short transverse central ridging due to habit tic; toes spared
Serial	Often manicure-induced, toes usually spared
Paronychia	Mostly lateral nail plate affected, often with discoloration due to bacterial colonization
Runaround	Only affected finger involved, sometimes onychomadesis

■■■ MECHANICAL, CHEMICAL, AND PHYSICAL CAUSES

Nail biting (Figure 1.42) is a frequent cause of an irregular nail surface and nail dystrophy. The mechanical trauma repeatedly injures the matrix, causing disturbances of nail formation. In extreme cases, this may lead to complete nail loss.

Habitual picking of a nail (Figure 1.43), usually one or both thumbnails, is done either with the index fingernail of the same hand when only one nail is involved, or with the thumbnail of the other hand in more or less symmetrical involvement of both thumbnails. Commonly, it is the central part of the nail that exhibits a washboard-like appearance.[66] This condition is often misdiagnosed as median central dystrophy of Heller. In most cases, the cuticle is pushed

■ TABLE 1.7

Associations of Reil–Beau lines

Systemic disease	Local
Febrile disease	Chronic skin disease:
Infectious diseases:	• Paronychia, eczema
• Typhus, acute rheumatic fever, diphtheria, syphilis, parotitis, malaria, gonococcal arthritis, scarlet fever, epididymitis (Beau's original description was in typhoid and other systemic disorders)	• Pustular psoriasis • Pemphigus foliaceus
• Erythema nodosum leprosum (recurrent attacks, multiple Reil–Beau lines)	Trauma: • Traumatic: overzealous manicure, neurotic cuticle-pushing ('washboard nails')
• Mucocutaneous lymph node syndrome	• Hand trauma
• Acquired immunodeficiency syndrome (AIDS)	• Fractured and immobilized wrist
Severe carential states (proteins, vitamins, pellagra)	Carpal tunnel syndrome (ischemic skin lesions, acro-osteolysis, and thickened dystrophic nails with Reil–Beau lines)
Circulatory:	
• Myocardial infarction	
• Peripheral vascular disease accompanied by arteriolar obliteration, Raynaud's disease	
• Pulmonary embolism	
• Prolonged tourniquet at surgery affecting all the digits on that limb	
Dysmetabolic states (in particular, diabetes, hypothyroidism, hypocalcemia, hypoparathyroidism)	
Sheehan syndrome (hypopituitarism)	
Digestive diseases: diarrhea, chronic enterocolitis, subacute and chronic pancreatitis with malabsorption syndrome, sprue, severe gastritis, acrodermatitis enteropathica	
Drugs:	
• Dapsone, retinoids, carbamazepine, razoxane and other chemotherapeutic agents	
Erythroderma:	
• If due to drugs: 'shoreline nails'	

■ TABLE 1.7

Associations of Reil–Beau lines (*continued*)

Systemic disease	Local
Surgery	
Chronic alcoholism, arsenic toxicity	
Strong emotional disturbance, especially if prolonged, hysteria, post epileptic convulsions	
Gynecologic: • Parturition; in the newborn period associated with traumas of pregnancy or parturition (more frequent following forceps delivery), • Dysmenorrhea	
Congenital: Can appear at 1 month of age and grow out by 4 months	

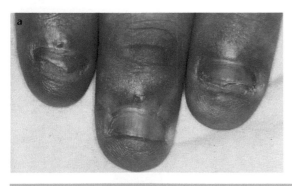 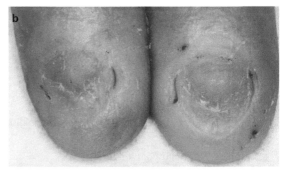

■ FIGURE 1.42 (a,b)

Nail biting.

back so that the thumbnail elongates. When the blind end of the proximal groove is exposed by this habit, there is malformation of the dorsal layer of the nail (which is responsible for the nail shine), resulting in the nail becoming dull. Manipulating the cuticle and proximal nail fold is an isolated habit. Habitual picking and nail biting are more frequent in persons with obsessive–compulsive disorders as well as their healthy relatives than in control subjects without impulse control disorders.

Typically, after an operation on the nail or after nail avulsion, a transverse depression appears that runs parallel to the lunula.

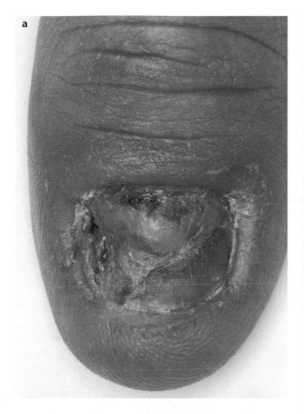

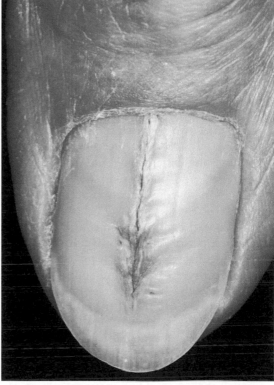

■ FIGURE 1.44
Heller's dystrophia unguis mediana canaliformis.

■ FIGURE 1.43

(a) Habitual picking. (b) Pushing back of the cuticle, exhibiting a washboard-like appearance.

Dystrophia unguis mediana canaliformis (Figure 1.44) was described by Heller in 1928. It may be characterized by a series of densely arranged parallel transverse ridges of approximately 2.5 mm running in the center of the nail from the cuticle to the free margin and causing a slight canaliform depression. Another type exhibits a central split, from which oblique narrow grooves run proximally. The cause of this condition is not known, although trauma, especially repeated pressure on the base of the nail, has been suggested.[67]

Scratches on the nail surface may be a professional stigma of tailors.

Distal triangular worn-down nails have recently been described.[68,69]

Nail changes due to accidental or professional **X-ray exposure** were described as early as the end of the 19th century. The nails may lose their shine and develop roughness, longitudinal ridges, brittleness, and melanotic streaks.[70] **Radiation treatment** may also cause a dull, lusterless, somewhat opaque nail. The tip of the finger may be involved and may aid in the diagnosis with typical radiodermatitis changes.

Longstanding contact with a number of **chemicals**, especially aggressive alkaline substances and salt solutions, causes the nails to swell and to become whitish and rough. Long-term application of nail varnish, leaving it on and applying layer upon layer, causes a dull and soft surface and whitish spots called nail granulations. Caustic alkaline substances used to remove the cuticle may enter under the proximal nail fold and impair the most proximal matrix, with consequent damage to the dorsal nail layer.

In addition to the other characteristics of the condition, **onychogrypotic nails** also have an irregular surface, which presents commonly with transverse ridges and splits. Opaque, discolored nails with an oyster-shell-like surface are seen in **congenital malalignment** of the big toenails[71,72] (Figure 1.45).

Age-related changes of the nail surface include **herringbone nails** in children[73,74] (Figure 1.46) and **longitudinal ridging**, often with beading, in elderly persons[75] (Figure 1.47). Interestingly, linear rows of drops of wax-like elevations have been observed in psoriasis[76] (Figure 1.48).

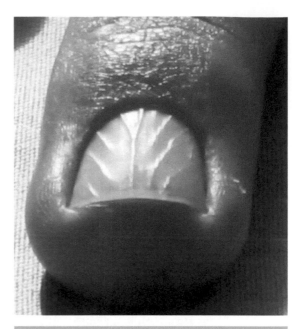

■ FIGURE 1.46
Herringbone nail in a child.

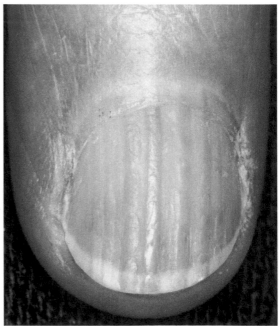

■ FIGURE 1.47
Longitudinal ridging with beading in an elderly person.

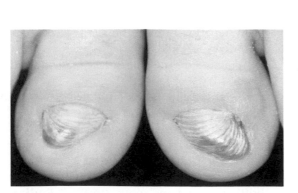

■ FIGURE 1.45
Oyster-shell-like surface in congenital malalignment.

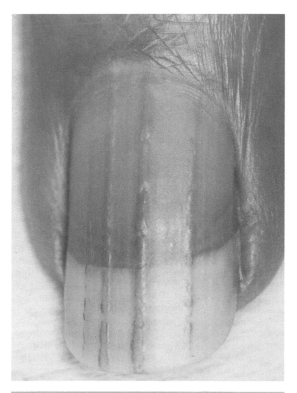

Psoriatic linear rows of drops of wax-like elevations.

■■■ REFERENCES

1. Kumar B, Jain R, Sandhu K, Kaur I, Handa S. Epidemiology of childhood psoriasis: a study of 419 patients from northern India. Int J Dermatol 2004; 43: 654–8.
2. Scheinfeld NS. Trachyonychia: a case report and review of manifestations, associations, and treatments. Cutis 2003; 71: 299–302.
3. Beau JHS. Note sure certains caractères de séméiologie rétrospective présentés par les ongles. Arch Gén Méd 1846; 11: 447.
4. Eastmond CJ, Wright V. The nail dystrophy of psoriatic arthritis. Ann Rheum Dis 1979; 38: 226–8.
5. Lovy M, Bluhm G, Morales A. The occurrence of pitting in Reiter's syndrome. J Am Acad Dermatol 1980; 2: 66–8.
6. Pajarre R, Kero M. Nail changes as the first manifestation of the HLA-B27 inheritance. A case report. Dermatologica 1977; 154: 350–4.
7. Nnoruka EN. Current epidemiology of atopic dermatitis in south-eastern Nigeria. Int J Dermatol 2004; 43: 739–44.
8. Hemmer W, Focke M, Wantke F, Götz M, Jarisch R. Allergic contact dermatitis to artificial fingernails prepared from UV light-cured acrylates. J Am Acad Dermatol 1996; 35: 377–80.
9. Tan E, Tay YK, Goh CL, Chin Giam Y. The pattern and profile of alopecia areata in Singapore – a study of 219 Asians. Int J Dermatol 2002; 41: 748–51.
10. Nanda A, Al-Fouzan AS, Al-Hasawi F. Alopecia areata in children: a clinical profile. Pediatr Dermatol 2002; 19: 482–5.
11. Samman PD. Trachyonychia (rough nails). Br J Dermatol 1979; 101: 701–5.
12. Baran R, Dawber R. Cutis. Twenty-nail dystrophy of childhood: a misnamed syndrome. Cutis 1987; 39: 481–2.
13. Baran R. Twenty nail dystrophy of alopecia areata. Arch Dermatol 1981; 117: 1.
14. Braun-Falco O, Dorn M, Neubert U, Plewig G. Trachyonychia: 20-nail dystrophy. Hautarzt 1981; 32: 17–22.
15. Taniguchi S, Kutsuna H, Tani Y, Kawahira K, Hamada T. Twenty-nail dystrophy (trachyonychia) caused by lichen planus in a patient with alopecia universalis and ichthyosis vulgaris. J Am Acad Dermatol 1995; 33: 903–5.
16. Jerasutus S, Suvanprakorn P, Kitchawengkul O. Twenty-nail dystrophy. A clinical manifestation of spongiotic inflammation of the nail matrix. Arch Dermatol 1990; 126: 1068–70.
17. Tosti A, Bardazzi F, Piraccini BM, Fanti PA. Idiopathic trachyonychia (twenty-nail dystrophy): a pathological study of 23 patients. Br J Dermatol 1994; 131: 866–72.
18. Alkiewicz J, Górny W. Zur Klinik und Histopathologie der Längsfurchen der menschlichen Nagelplatte. Arch Derm Syph (Berl) 1937; 175: 467–75.
19. Peluso AM, Tosti A, Piraccini BM, Cameli N. Lichen planus limited to the nails in childhood: case report and literature review. Pediatr Dermatol 1993; 10: 36–9.
20. Takeuchi Y, Iwase N, Suzuki M, Tsuyuki S. Lichen planus with involvement of all twenty nails and the oral mucous membrane. J Dermatol 2000; 27: 94–8.
21. Scott MJ Jr, Scott MJ Sr. Ungual lichen planus. Lichen planus of the nail. Arch Dermatol 1979; 115: 1197–9.
22. Samman PD. The nails in lichen planus. Br J Dermatol 1961; 73: 288–92.
23. Cram DL, Kierland RR, Winkelmann RK. Ulcerative lichen planus of the feet. Bullous variant with hair and nail lesions. Arch Dermatol 1966; 93: 692–701.
24. Samman PD. Idiopathic atrophy of the nails. Br J Dermatol 1969; 81: 746–9.
25. Zaias N. The nail in lichen planus. Arch Dermatol 1970; 101: 264–71.
26. Cornelius CE 3rd, Shelley WB. Permanent anonychia due to lichen planus. Arch Dermatol 1967; 96: 434–5.
27. Haneke E. Isolated bullous lichen planus of the nails mimicking yellow nail syndrome. Clin Exp Dermatol 1983; 8: 425–8.
28. Fanti PA, Tosti A, Morelli R, Galbiati G. Nail changes as the first sign of systemic amyloidosis. Dermatologica 1991; 183: 44–6.
29. Mancuso G, Fanti PA, Berdondini RM. Nail changes as the only skin abnormality in myeloma-associated systemic amyloidosis. Br J Dermatol 1997; 137: 471–2.
30. Pineda MS, Herrero C, Palou J, Vilalta A, Mascaró JM. Nail alterations in systemic amyloidosis: report of one case, with histologic study. J Am Acad Dermatol 1988; 18: 1357–9.

31. Baran R, Dupré A, Lauret P, Puissant A. Lichen striatus with nail involvement. Report of 4 cases and review of the 4 cases in the literature. Ann Dermatol Venereol 1979; 106: 885–91.

32. Laugier P, Olmos L. Naevus linéaire inflammatoire et lichen striatus. Deux aspects d'une même affection. Bull Soc Fr Derm Syph 1976; 83: 48–53.

33. Bazex A, Griffiths WAD. Acrokeratosis paraneoplastica. A new cutaneous marker of malignancy. Br J Dermatol 1980; 102: 304.

34. Bolognia JL, Brewer YP, Cooper DL. Bazex syndrome (acrokeratosis paraneoplastica). An analytic review. Medicine (Baltimore) 1991; 70: 269–80.

35. Haneke E, Djawari D: Hyperimmunglobulin E-Syndrom: Atopisches Ekzem, Eosinophilie, Chemotaxisdefekt, Infektanfälligkeit und chronische mucocutane Candidose. Akt Dermatol 1982; 8: 34–9.

36. Haneke E. Fungal infections of the nail. Semin Dermatol 1991; 10: 41–53.

37. Fritsch P. Lichen nitidus (Pinkus). Z Haut Geschlechtskr 1967; 42: 649–66.

38. Kellett JK, Beck MH. Lichen nitidus associated with distinctive nail changes. Clin Exp Dermatol 1984; 9: 201–4.

39. Sonnex TS, Dawber RP, Zachary CB, Millard PR, Griffiths AD. The nails in adult type 1 pityriasis rubra pilaris. A comparison with Sézary syndrome and psoriasis. J Am Acad Dermatol 1986; 15: 956–60.

40. Lambert DG, Dalac S. Nail changes in type V pityriasis rubra pilaris. J Am Acad Dermatol 1989; 21: 118–21.

41. Kocsard E. The dystrophic nail of keratotic scabies. Am J Dermatopathol 1984; 6: 308–9.

42. Witkowski JA, Parish LC. Scabies. Subungual areas harbor mites. JAMA 1984; 252: 1318–19.

43. Hjorth N, Thomsen K. Parakeratosis pustulosa. Br J Dermatol 1967; 79: 527–32.

44. Botella R, Martinez C, Albero P, Mascaro JM. Parakeratosis pustolosa de Hjorth. Discusión nosológica a propósito de tres casos. Acta Dermato-Sifil 1973; 1–2: 101.

45. Tosti A, Peluso AM, Zucchelli V. Clinical features and long-term follow-up of 20 cases of parakeratosis pustulosa. Pediatr Dermatol 1998; 15: 259–63.

46. Zaias N, Ackerman AB. The nail in Darier–White disease. Arch Dermatol 1973; 107: 193–9.

47. Cooper SM, Burge SM. Darier's disease: epidemiology, pathophysiology, and management. Am J Clin Dermatol 2003; 4: 97–105.

48. Burge SM. Hailey–Hailey disease: the clinical features, response to treatment and prognosis. Br J Dermatol 1992; 126: 275–82.

49. Gao XH, Li X, Zhao Y, Wang Y, Chen HD. Familial koilonychia. Int J Dermatol 2001; 40: 290–1.

50. Gupta R, Mehta S, Pandhi D, Singal A. Hereditary punctate palmoplantar keratoderma (PKK) (Brauer–Buschke–Fischer syndrome). J Dermatol 2004; 31: 398–402.

51. Tosti A, Morelli R, Fanti PA, Cameli N. Nail changes of punctate keratoderma: a clinical and pathological study of two patients. Acta Derm Venereol 1993; 73: 66–8.

52. Combemale P, Kanitakis J. Epidermolysis bullosa simplex with mottled pigmentation. Case report and review of the literature. Dermatology 1994; 189: 173–8.

53. Garman ME, Nunez-Gussman J, Metry D. What syndrome is this? Keratosis follicularis spinulosa decalvans. Ped Dermatol 2005; 22: 170–4.

54. Baden HP, Byers HR. Clinical findings, cutaneous pathology, and response to therapy in 21 patients with keratosis pilaris atrophicans. Arch Dermatol 1994; 130: 469–75.

55. Sato-Matsumura KC, Matsumura T, Kumakiri M Tsuji Y, Ohkawara A. Ichthyosis follicularis with alopecia and photophobia in a mother and daughter. Br J Dermatol 2000; 142: 157–62.

56. Nieves DS, Phipps RP, Pollock SJ, et al. Dermatologic and immunologic findings in the immune dysregulation, polyendocrinopathy, enteropathy, X-linked syndrome. Arch Dermatol 2004; 140: 466–72.

57. Janjua SA, Khachemoune A. Papillon–Lefèvre syndrome: a case report and review of the literature. Dermatol Online J 2004; Jul 15,10(1): 13.

58. Pollak C, Floy M, Say B. Sensorineural hearing loss and enamel hypoplasia with subtle nail findings: another family with Heimler's syndrome. Clin Dysmorphol 2003; 12: 55–8.

59. Yashiro M, Kobayashi H, Kubo N, et al. Cronkhite–Canada syndrome containing colon cancer and serrated adenoma lesions. Digestion 2004; 69: 57–62.

60. Kalb RE, Grossman ME. Pterygium formation due to sarcoidosis. Arch Dermatol 1985; 121: 276–7.

61. Cox HN, Gawkrodger DJ. Nail dystrophy in chronic sarcoidosis. Br J Dermatol 1988; 118: 697–701.

62. Mallinson CN, Bloom SR, Warin P. A glucagonoma syndrome. Lancet 1974; ii: 1–5.

63. Haneke E. Nagelveränderungen bei Erkrankungen des Endokriniums. Therapiewoche 1987; 37: 4379–82.

64. Fabry H. Gleichzeitiges rhythmisches Auftreten von Querfurchen der Nägel und gruppierten Knotenbildungen der Haare. Z Haut-GeschlKr 1965; 39: 336–8.

65. Kaur I, Chakrabarti A, Dogra S, Rai R, Kumar B. Nail involvement in leprosy: a study of 300 patients. Int J Lepr Other Mycobact Dis 2003; 71: 320–7.

66. McAulay WL. Transverse ridging of the thumbnails – 'washboard thumbnails'. Arch Dermatol 1966; 93: 421–32.

67. Teller H, Thal M. Zur Klinik und Pathogenese der Dystrophia unguium mediana canaliformis. Dermatol Wschr 1958; 137: 380–6.

68. Baran R, Moulin G. The bidet nail: a French variant of the worn-down syndrome. Br J Dermatol 1999; 140: 377.

69. Piraccini BM, Tullo S, Iorizzo M. Triangular worn-down nails: report of 14 cases. G Ital Dermatol Venereol 2005; 140: 261–4.

70. Richert B, de la Brassinne M. Subungual chronic radiodermatis. Dermatology 1993; 186: 290–3.

71. Baran R, Bureau H. Congenital malalignment of the big toenail as a cause of ingrowing toenail in infancy. Pathology and treatment (a study of thirty cases). Clin Exp Dermatol 1983; 8: 619–23.

72. Baran R, Haneke E. Etiology and treatment of nail malalignment. Dermatol Surg 1998; 24: 719–21.

73. Parry EJ, Morley WN, Dawber RPR. Herringbone nails: an uncommon variant of nail growth in childhood? Br J Dermatol 1995; 132: 1021–2.

74. Shuster S. The significance of chevron nails. Br J Dermatol 1996; 135: 144–61.

75. Helfand AE. Nail and hyperkeratotic problems in the elderly foot. Am Fam Phys 1989; 39: 101–10.

76. Baden HP. Nail abnormalities associated with cutaneous disease. In: Diseases of Hair and Nails. Chicago: Year Book, 1987: 49.

Chapter 2

Severe nail dystrophy, hyponychia and anonychia, and alterations of nail shape

▪▪▪ DERMATOLOGICAL DISEASES

All types of nail dystrophies, in addition to most of the under surface alterations described in Chapter 1, may progress to severe atrophy and eventually anonychia.

Psoriasis vulgaris, particularly **psoriatic arthritis** with lesions of the periungual skin, often causes severe nail dystrophy (Figure 2.1). This is due to matrix involvement that is continuous from the dorsal and ventral surfaces of the proximal nail fold to the matrix. The nail becomes rough, crumbly, opaque, and discolored with an irregular surface, and will finally be reduced to keratotic debris.[1,2] The involvement of the dorsal and ventral surfaces of the proximal nail fold causes the cuticle to disappear, with consequent detachment of the nail plate from the eponychium, and dirt, foreign bodies, and

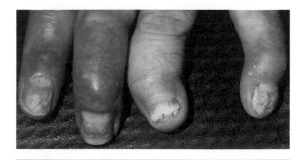

■ FIGURE 2.1

Psoriatic arthritis. (Courtesy of RE Kalb, USA.)

potential pathogens may be trapped under the nail fold and exacerbate the disease. When the distal interphalangeal joint is affected, it is usually swollen and often stiff in a slight flexion of 160°–170°. The distal phalanx itself often appears to be shorter and/or slightly tapered.

There are different types of **pustular psoriasis** of the nail organ. First, the nail may be involved in the course of **generalized psoriasis pustulosa of von Zumbusch**, where some subungual small yellow spots may be seen reflecting pustules of the nail bed. As this is usually an acute condition, they do not commonly cause a severe nail dystrophy. Also in the course of **palmoplantar pustular psoriasis of Königsbeck**, nail involvement with subungual pustules can occur and deep erosions of the nail plate can be observed. The pustules tend to be more chronic than those of the generalized form, but usually do not lead to permanent nail dystrophy. In contrast, **acrodermatitis continua suppurativa of Hallopeau** (Figures 2.2 and 2.3) is an insidious, extremely chronic, and progressive acropustulosis that often involves only one nail and remains undiagnosed for a long period of time. However, many nails may become affected. Typically, and in contrast to other forms of psoriasis and acropustuloses, it remains confined to the nail region,[3] although classical psoriatic lesions are sometimes seen elsewhere – far away from the nails – on the body or extremities. The disease starts with painless pustules under and/or around the nail that consistently

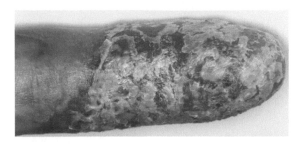

■ FIGURE 2.2
Acrodermatitis continua suppurativa.

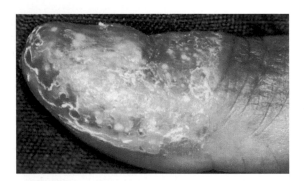

■ FIGURE 2.3
Acrodermatitis continua suppurativa.

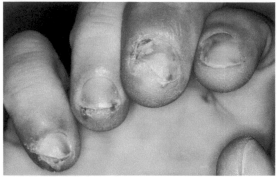

■ FIGURE 2.4
Reiter syndrome.

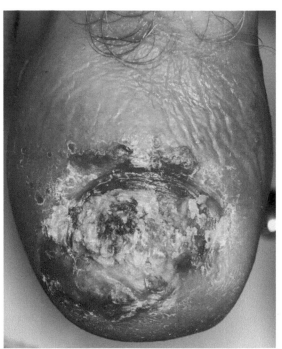

■ FIGURE 2.5
Reiter syndrome.

recur and slowly destroy the entire nail. Even the distal digit may be lost.[4] Treatment is notoriously recalcitrant. Many new drugs have been tried, but have mostly been found to be ineffective. Whether or not new biological agents will usher in a new era in the treatment of this disease remains to be seen.

Histologically, three different types of acral pustular psoriasis are seen: a spongiform pustular type as seen in typical pustular psoriasis of the skin, an eczematous spongiotic type, and a mixed type.

In **Reiter syndrome** virtually identical alterations of the nail (Figure 2.4) and the distal phalanx including the joints are seen (Figure 2.5). Nail lesions are commonly more severe in Reiter syndrome with ungual involvement, and a hemorrhagic component may give them a brownish tinge. As in psoriasis, almost complete nail dys-

trophy with severe deformation of the nail keratin develops, particularly in cases where onset has been acute.

The classical example of severe nail dystrophy with eventual sclero-atrophy (Figure 2.6) of the nail field is **nail lichen planus**, which may

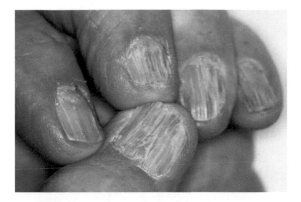

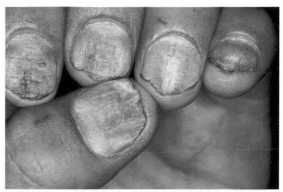

■ **FIGURE 2.6**

Nail ridging in lichen planus.

■ **FIGURE 2.7**

Lichen planus sandpaper nail dystrophy.

start with ridged nails (Figure 2.7), sandpapered nail dystrophy, ulceration of the nail field, pterygium formation, and finally more or less complete loss of the nail.[5,6] The fingertip may then present with a smooth dorsal surface of the distal phalanx. Particularly in ulcerating lichen planus of the distal phalanx – a rare form seen mainly on the toes – severe scarring may be obvious.

Total dystrophic onychomycosis is by definition associated with severe to complete nail dystrophy (Figure 2.8). Except for chronic mucocutaneous candidosis, where this is a primary event,[7] cases due to dermatophytes and molds commonly develop from distal subungual onychomycosis, and much less frequently from proximal subungual, endonyx, or superficial white onychomycosis. The patient's history will give valuable information about the diagnosis. Usually, not all nails are affected. The nail may be split into several parts, onycholytic, discolored, brittle, or reduced to keratotic debris. The last of these is typical of chronic mucocutaneous candidosis. Chronic mucocutaneous candidosis may also be associated with hypothyroidism or a polyendocrinopathy.

Severe nail destruction can be observed in **chilblain lupus** (Figure 2.9), whereas gangrene of the digital tips may occur in **systemic lupus erythematosus (SLE)**[8,9] (Figure 2.10). However,

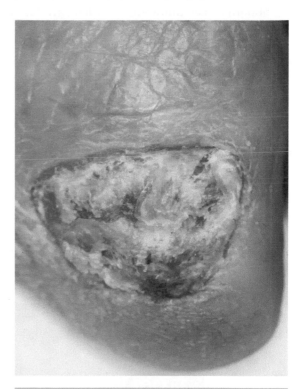

■ **FIGURE 2.8**

Total dystrophic onychomycosis.

none of these changes allow a diagnosis of lupus erythematosus to be made without other skin lesions or histopathology. Other changes seen in lupus erythematosus are splinter hemorrhages,

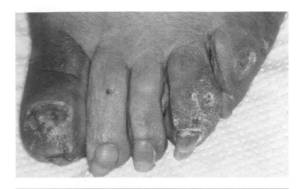

■ FIGURE 2.9

Chilblain lupus.

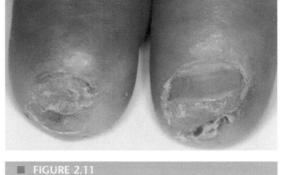

■ FIGURE 2.11

Acral scleroderma.

abnormal keratinization with leukonychia, red lunulae, pitting, ridging, Reil–Beau lines, onycholysis, and onychomadesis. Additionally, clubbing and pterygium inversum have been observed. In Black patients, longitudinal brown streaks or a blue–black nail coloration may be seen, reflecting either activation of melanocytes or pigmentary incontinence. Mutilating acral lupus erythematosus has also been observed.[10]

Complete loss of several toenails as the only cutaneous sign has been observed in a case of **dermatomyositis.**[11]

In the **acral type of scleroderma**, the tip of the digit may be slowly resorbed and the nail may finally become hypoplastic (Figure 2.11) until it disappears completely, usually together with considerable resorption of the terminal phalanx, finally leaving only a narrow crescent of bone adjacent to the distal interphalangeal joint.[12]

Pemphigus vulgaris may involve the nails and cause complete loss of affected nails. Ungual involvement is more common on finger- than toenails and is mostly restricted to severe forms of pemphigus although this has recently been disputed. An analysis of 64 patients with pemphigus vulgaris revealed nail changes in almost half.[13] It commonly starts with lesions reminiscent of subacute to chronic paronychia (Figure 2.12) or even warts, trachyonychia, Reil–Beau lines and deeper transverse grooves, and lead to onychomadesis (Figure 2.13). Multiple subun-

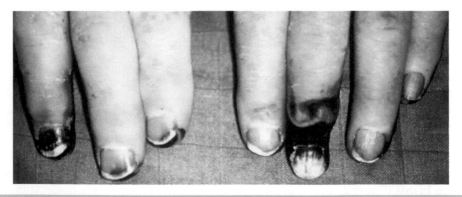

■ FIGURE 2.10

Systemic lupus erythematosus.

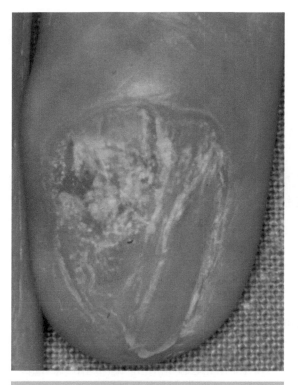

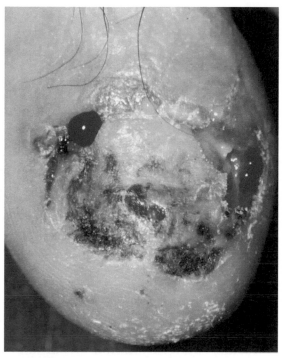

■ FIGURE 2.14

Nail shedding in pemphigus vulgaris.

■ FIGURE 2.12

Subacute paronychia in pemphigus vulgaris.

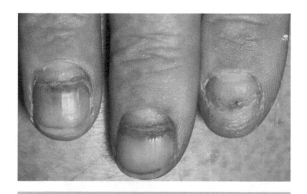

■ FIGURE 2.13

Onychomadesis in pemphigus vulgaris.

gual hematomas followed by onychomadesis have been reported in one case. Nail shedding may be observed in primary nail bed pemphigus (Figure 2.14). Histopathology shows suprabasal

acantholytic blister formation with the typical immunofluorescence pattern of intercellular immunoglobulin G (IgG) and complement component 3 (C3) deposition.

Vegetating pemphigus of Hallopeau may clinically resemble acrodermatitis continua suppurativa with sterile pustules and complete nail atrophy[14,15] (Figure 2.15).

Nail shedding, in addition to yellowish nail discoloration, onychorrhexis, and onycholysis, may occur in **Brazilian pemphigus (fogo selvagem)**.[16]

Blistering in the course of **bullous pemphigoid** is comparable to that of normal skin, as the nail has the same basement membrane antigens. However, in severe cases, the blistering may lead to nail loss,[17] whereas less severe involvement causes transverse lines. Periungual blistering is not rare. Immunofluorescence reveals IgM and C3 at the basement membrane.

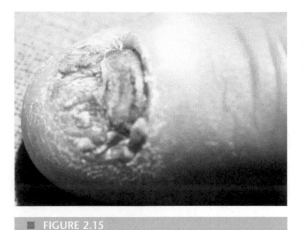

■ FIGURE 2.15

Vegetating pemphigus.

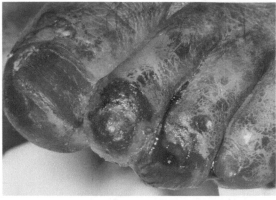

■ FIGURE 2.16

Nail loss in Lyell syndrome.

Severe nail dystrophy with ridging and splits[18] has been seen in **cicatricial pemphigoid**.

Depending on the severity of matrix and nail bed attack by the disease, **erythema multiforme, Stevens–Johnson syndrome** and **Lyell syndrome** may lead to onychomadesis, complete nail loss (Figure 2.16), and pterygium formation. This may be an acute event, or a severely dystrophic nail may grow out from under the proximal nail fold (Figure 2.17). Blistering diseases may also mimic paronychia and lead secondarily to nail changes.

Epidermolysis bullosa acquisita, a rare immunobullous dermatosis, may cause onycholysis and nail loss.[19]

Chronic erythroderma of whatever cause usually leads to progressive alopecia and atrophy of the nails, beginning with loss of nail shine and transparency, brittleness, and surface roughness[20] (Figure 2.18). Later, the nails may fall off, or just disappear insidiously and almost completely.

A variety of **subungual tumors** may lead to nail dystrophy and finally nail loss. This is the

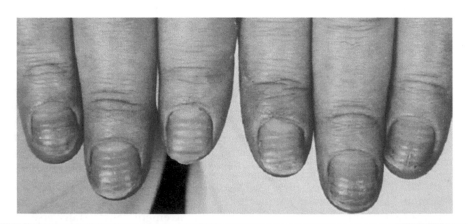

■ FIGURE 2.17

Transverse lines associated with chemotherapy. (Courtesy of PHTJ Slee, The Netherlands.)

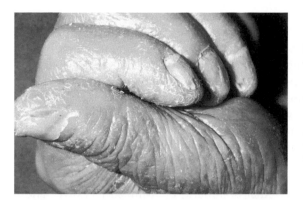

Onychomadesis in chronic erythroderma.

case not only when the matrix is involved, but also when there is extensive nail bed involvement or there is a large bulging tumor mass.

■■■ SYSTEMIC CONDITIONS

Marked nail dystrophy of all fingernails may occur in **systemic amyloidosis**[21] (Figure 2.19). Chronic **hemodialysis** causes a self-limited bullous pseudoporphyria hemodialytica. Severe photo-onycholysis with loss of the nails and ulceration of the nail beds has been observed.[22] Reversible pseudoclubbing of all fingernails, followed by onychomadesis, has been described in a **peritoneal dialysis** patient two months after *Acinetobacter peritonitis* infection.

Calciphylaxis in renal insufficiency and renal transplant patients as well as those undergoing long-term dialysis is known to cause necrosis that may involve the tips of the fingers and/or toes. Depending on the extent of the necrosis (Figure 2.20), nail dystrophy or loss will develop.[23]

Peripheral neuropathy with acro-osteolysis can also cause digital tip necrosis with loss of the nail. In the acquired form, which is usually due to alcohol abuse or diabetes mellitus, this may lead to an enormous enlargement of

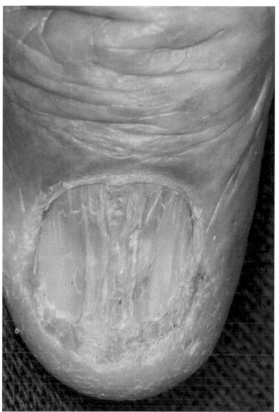

Systemic amyloidosis.

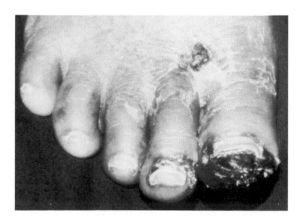

Calciphylaxis. (Courtesy of P Chang, Guatemala.)

the terminal phalanx, with an associated increase in the size of the nail.

Leprosy is another cause of severe nail dystrophy and nail loss. However, it is not the mycobacterial infection itself, but rather the leprotic neuropathy and the concomitant and subsequent unnoticed repeated trauma that is the cause of these severe nail lesions.[24] Asymmetrical nail dystrophy and anonychia may be observed in **syringomyelia**.[25]

■■■ GENETIC DISEASES

Nail dystrophy of various morphological types is a component of all **ectodermal dysplasias** with nail involvement. Of the almost 200 different ectodermal dysplasias that have so far been described, the hidrotic tricho-onychotic type of Clouston is the most common.[26] The nails may exhibit a fluting that increases distally, may be flat or spoon-shaped, and may be brittle. Anonychia has also been observed in a case of autosomal dominant ectrodactyly syndrome.

Lelis syndrome (ectodermal dysplasia with acanthosis nigricans) is characterized by nail dystrophy, hypotrichosis, hypohidrosis, palmoplantar hyperkeratosis, early-onset loss of permanent teeth, mental retardation, and acanthosis nigricans.

Progressive nail dystrophy is seen in the autosomal recessive **skin fragility–ectodermal dysplasia syndrome** due to mutations in the plakophilin 1 gene. It is otherwise characterized by skin and hair defects of varying degree.

Dyskeratosis congenita is characterized by nail dystrophy, reticular pigmentation of the skin, leukoplakia of the oral mucosa, pancytopenia, immunodeficiency, and an increased tendency to develop malignant tumors even at an early age. It may be autosomal recessive, autosomal dominant, or X-linked recessive. The nails become thin, often slightly ridged, and tend to split[27] (Figures 2.21 and 2.22).

Nail dystrophy is a common feature of the severe cicatricial forms of **epidermolysis bullosa hereditaria**, being most pronounced in the dystrophic form of Hallopeau–Siemens. Blistering from minor trauma also involves the nail organ, and leads to nail dystrophy and finally complete scarring of the former nail field. However, toenail dystrophy has also been observed in pretibial dystrophic epidermolysis bullosa.[28] In **junctional epidermolysis bullosa (JEB)**, painful nail dystrophy is typical at the beginning, while later in the course of the disease, thick layers of former blister roofs accumulate under the nail, mimicking subungual hyperkeratosis. Nail changes are identical in generalized benign atrophic epidermolysis bullosa.[29]

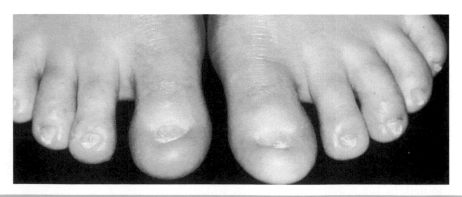

■ **FIGURE 2.21**

Dyskeratosis congenita. (Courtesy of CG Schirren, Germany.)

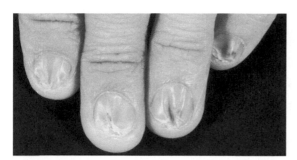

■ FIGURE 2.22

Dyskeratosis congenita. (Courtesy of E Blume-Peytavi, Germany.)

Complete anonychia may develop[30] (Figures 2.23 and 2.24). Junctional epidermolyses are due to mutations in the genes encoding the hemidesmosome-anchoring filament complex proteins, laminin 5, and the 180 kDa bullous pemphigoid antigen.

The nail changes in **laryngo-onycho-cutaneous syndrome (Shabbir syndrome)** resemble those of junctional epidermolysis bullosa, and in fact both are due to a defect in the α_3 chain of laminin 5; this chain is completely lacking in JEB, whereas only the portion docking to the dermal part of the basement membrane complex is lacking in Shabbir syndrome. Ultimately, the nails are lost in both laminin 5

defect syndromes. Of the simplex forms, the **herpetiform type of Dowling–Meara** presents nail dystrophy. Autosomal recessive **epidermolysis bullosa hereditaria simplex with neuromuscular involvement** may also develop nail dystrophy in association with atrophic scarring, scalp alopecia, milia formation, and oral mucosal lesions.

Congenital bullous poikiloderma (Kindler syndrome)[31] is an autosomal recessive skin fragility syndrome with photosensitivity and acral blistering in infancy followed by progressive poikiloderma and mucocutaneous scarring. It is due to loss-of-function mutations in a novel gene on chromosome 20p12.3, *KIND1*, encoding kindlin-1, which is produced in basal keratinocytes and is involved in the attachment of the intracellular actin cytoskeleton to the extracellular matrix. Nail dystrophy in the course of this rare disease has been observed in two cases.

Congenital homolateral epidermal hyperplasia or hypoplastic hemidysplasia (CHILD syndrome) of Happle may cause grotesque nail dystrophy that is confined to the side of the main pathology[32] (Figure 2.25).

■ ■ ■ PHYSICAL, MECHANICAL, AND CHEMICAL INJURY

Longstanding use of the nails as a tool for mechanical work causes wearing and loss of the

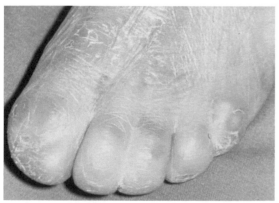

■ FIGURE 2.23

Generalized benign atrophic epidermolysis bullosa. (Courtesy of I Anton Lamprecht, Germany.)

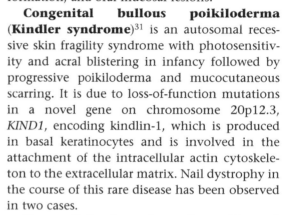

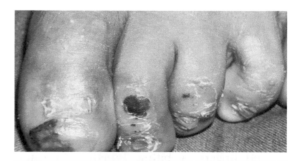

■ FIGURE 2.24

Epidermolysis bullosa.

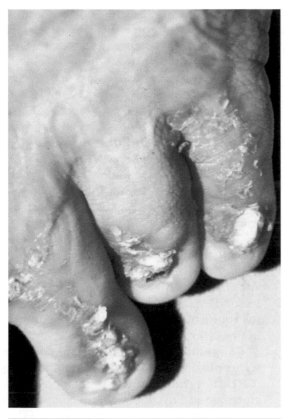

CHILD syndrome. (Courtesy of G Moulin, France.)

free margin of the nail plate as seen in **fly-tier's nail**, in tailors, etc.

Autodestructive habits such as nail biting, onychophagia, onychotillomania, and ony-chotemnomania can cause severe nail dystrophy up to temporary or even permanent anonychia. This is also seen in syndromes where patients do not feel pain (as in leprosy and syringomyelia). Biting of the fingertips is the cause for nail destruction and loss in **Lesch–Nyhan syndrome**, an X-linked inborn disease of uric acid metabolism with hyperuricemia, mental retardation, spastic cerebal palsy, choreoathetosis, and compulsive self-destruction of the lips, hands, and fingers by biting. Whether the causative defect in hypoxanthine–guanine phosphoribo-syltransferase is also responsible for effect on

presynaptic dopaminergic nerve terminals remains to be proven.

Laceration and crush injuries also cause nail deformation, dystrophy, or loss, depending on the severity of the trauma.

Nail loss may occur temporarily or permanently after **surgery** of the distal phalanx and even after **cryotherapy** (Figure 2.26).

Nail loss due to undetermined doses of **X-rays** was described soon after their discovery by Konrad Röntgen. The nails fell off, but regrew in some cases. More recent cases of radio-dermatitis, ranging from ridging, dullness, and opaqueness to partial and complete loss with scarring of the nail area have been described by many authors. They are now seldom seen due to the radioprotective measures that are generally imposed by health authorities. However, severe radiodermatitis of the nail area with skin and nail dystrophy, radiosclerosis, and telangiectasias is still seen in patients who, for instance, received X-irradiation for the treatment of common warts. The latency may be up to 25 years. Fortunately, radiation therapy of benign lesions is now exceptional.

More modern radiological treatment modalities can also cause loss of the nails. The nails fell off in patients who received total skin **electron-beam irradiation** for the treatment of mycosis

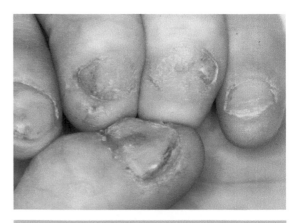

Permanent anonychia after cryotherapy.

fungoides: 48% of them experienced nail dystrophy after only 2000 cGy (Figure 2.27), whereas the nails were lost in 38% after the full dose of 3600 cGy. Intraarterial injection of 5-bromodeoxyuridine, a photoradiosensitizer used in the treatment of astrocytoma, caused nail loss in all patients. Transverse melanonychia has been reported with electron-beam irradiation.[33]

■■■ ALTERATIONS OF NAIL SHAPE

These changes concern the size, proportions and profile of the nail. It must be stressed here that they depend largely on the size and shape of the underlying bone of the terminal phalanx. In nail psoriasis, the nails may become shorter and/or wider, particularly in distal osteolysis of the terminal phalanx.[34] Psoriatic osteoarthropathy may cause a wider phalanx, with subsequent widening of the nail plate.

■■■ NAIL SIZE

Long nails are called **dolichonychia** (Figure 2.28). The length-to-width ratio is normally around 0.9–1.1; it is smaller in the thumb- and toenails than in the nails of the long fingers.

When this ratio is considerably greater, dolichonychia is diagnosed. It is commonly seen in **Marfan syndrome**, and sometimes also in **Ehlers–Danlos syndrome**.

Brachyonychia is diagnosed when the length-to-width ratio is considerably smaller than 0.9. It is common in persons with short stature. Brachyonychia also develops in patients who undergo long-term hemodialysis because of preterminal renal insufficiency and develop a tertiary hyperparathyroidism. In addition, the nail loses part of its tight connection with the rest of the underlying bone and can be easily moved to the sides and proximally.

Racket nails are short, wide nails due to a premature ossification of the epiphysis of the corresponding terminal phalanx, which from age 10–12 years onward no longer grows longitudinally but still becomes wider through apposition of bone. This leads to a characteristic racket shape of the entire distal phalanx. Most cases involve the thumbs symmetrically (Figure 2.29), although asymmetrical affection and involvement of other fingers and very rarely a toe may occur.[35]

A small nail – **micronychia** – is quite common on the little finger, often in association with clinodactyly (Figure 2.30).

Macronychia of all nails may be a sign of acromegaly. Single gigantic nails are seen in

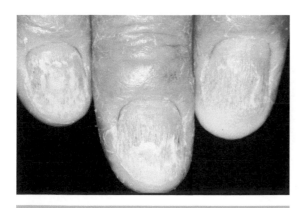

Nail dystrophy after electron-beam irradiation.

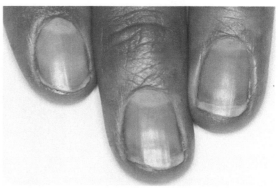

Dolichonychia.

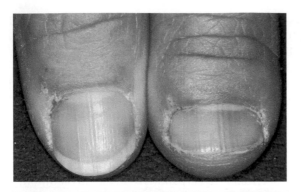

■ **FIGURE 2.29**

Racket nail.

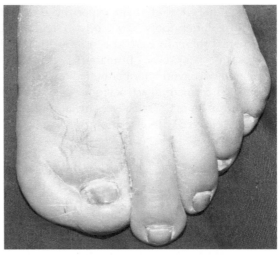

■ **FIGURE 2.30**

Micronychia. (Courtesy of P Chang, Guatemala.)

some rare malformation syndromes, with syndactyly when there is a synostosis of the terminal phalanx; this nail may look like one giant nail or present with a shallow longitudinal furrow indicating the fusion line of the underlying bone and the nail anlages. Very large nails, particularly on the big toe, can be seen in peripheral neuropathy with acro-osteolysis that leads to an enlargement of the involved terminal phalanx bone. Single-digit macronychia may occur in Proteus syndrome (Figure 2.31) and has also been described in patients with neurofibromatosis and epiloia. Hippocratic nails are also larger than normal (see below).

■■■ HYPONYCHIA AND ANONYCHIA

Hypoplasia and **aplasia of the nails** are probably only quantitative variations on the same underlying process and differ due to the time at which the development of the nail anlage was inhibited; some digits may exhibit hyponychia, some anonychia (Figure 2.32).

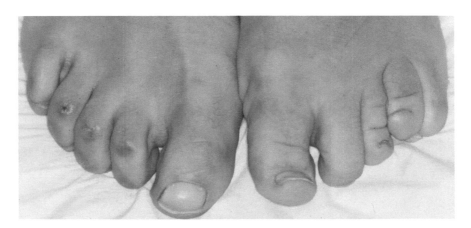

■ **FIGURE 2.31**

Macronychia.

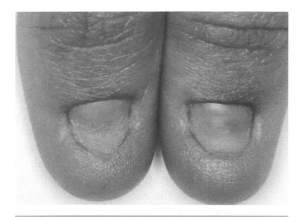

Congenital anonychia.

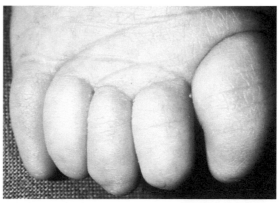

Cook syndrome. (Courtesy of D Eedy, UK.)

Four types of anyonychia are differentiated: **anonychia aplastica, anonychia atrophica solitaria, anonychia atrophica tarda,** and **anonychia keratodes.**

There have been a few cases of **hereditary anonychia**. A family of 10 afflicted members in three generations with **anonychia aplastica** of the ring finger, biphalangia, polydactyly, and joint damage was described by Alkiewicz.[36] These patients had a pit only in the centre of the tip of the digit, not on the dorsal aspect, which led the author to speculate that the nail anlage is primarily located in the axis of the finger and not on the dorsal aspect of the distal phalanx. Complete anonychia in monozygotic twins has recently been reported. Anonychia with microcephaly and normal intelligence was found in a consanguineous Iranian family. However, often the genetic background of anonychia is not elucidated.

In the case of **anonychia atrophica**, there is only keratotic material instead of a nail, and no real nail field is formed. Even already existing normal nails were observed to become scar tissue between the age of 5 and 8 years in two siblings.[36]

Zimmermann–Laband syndrome is characterized by gingival fibromatosis, aplastic or hypoplastic distal phalanges with koilonychia or absent nails, and enlargement of soft tissues of the face.

Four girls with **prepubertal gigantomastia and congenital anonychia** were described whose mothers both had normal breasts and normal nails, but whose fathers (who were related) also had congenital anonychia of the fingers and toes.

Many cases of anonychia also exhibit hypo- or aplasia of the terminal phalanx, as nail development depends on bone formation. The genetic defect in families with short fingers due to a congenital lack of the terminal phalanx and thus lack of nail development has recently been elucidated.

Cook syndrome (Figure 2.33) is characterized by absence of the terminal phalanges, hypoplasia of the first three fingernails, and anonychia on the ring and little fingers as well as the toes.[37]

A **syndrome of anonychia and deafness** is called the **DOOR syndrome**.

Nail–patella syndrome (hereditary onycho-osteodysplasia) (Figure 2.34) is due to a mutation of the *LMXB2* gene, which is responsible for anterior–posterior orientation during embryonic development and kidney development. Besides nail changes, a hypoplastic or completely lacking patella, iliac horns, severe nephropathy, and corneal alterations of the eyes may be present. Although there is considerable intrafamiliar variability, the expressivity of the disease is very

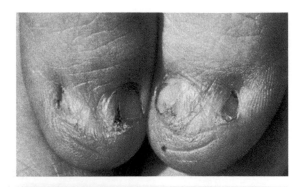

■ FIGURE 2.34

Nail–patella syndrome. (Courtesy of G Achten, Belgium.)

high. The nail matrix is usually triangular, and the nails may exhibit slight ridging, splits, hemiaplasia, or almost complete aplasia.[38] Normalization of the nail has been seen in a patient after successful renal transplantation.

Hypoplasia or hemiaplasia of the index finger is seen in **Iso–Kikuchi syndrome (congenital onychodysplasia of the index finger, COIF)**. The hypoplasia ranges from an only slightly smaller nail, to micronychia with deviation of the longitudinal axis, to hemionychia,[39] anonychia (Figure 2.35), micropolyonychia (Figure 2.36),

or hemionychogryposis. Sometimes, only a small piece of nail remains. This syndrome is inborn – not always hereditary, although one case with brachyphalangy and micronychia in the little toes of the father has been described. Unilateral or asymmetrical involvement is not uncommon. On X-ray films, a Y-shaped tip of the terminal phalanx is commonly seen. The nail changes are thought to be due to an impediment in the membranous ossification of the terminal phalanx, presumably caused by an ischemic process in utero. Malformation of the ear and involvement of the thumbs may occur, as well as a peculiar face and ear lobe malformations. Toenail involvement has been observed.

Nail dysplasia of the index fingers is also a sign of **sclerosteosis** characterized by asymmetrical syndactyly of the index and middle fingers. The syndrome, which is due to a nonmetabolic hyperactivity of osteoblasts, is very similar to van Buchem's disease, and both diseases map to the same chromosome region of 17q12–21. The osteoblast hyperactivity leads to obstruction of nerve canals and a large number of variable neurological abnormalities.[40]

Nail hypoplasia of the fifth finger is seen in **Coffin–Siris syndrome**, which is a complex developmental defect syndrome.[41]

Congenital anonychia is called **aplasia unguium**, and either occurs singly or may be

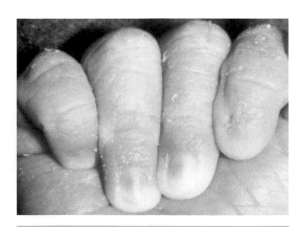

■ FIGURE 2.35

Anonychia in COIF (congenital onychodysplasia of the index finger) syndrome.

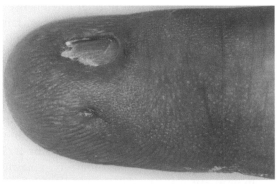

■ FIGURE 2.36

Micropolyonychia in COIF syndrome.

part of a complex malformation syndrome (e.g. DOOR syndrome) or a component of nail–patella syndrome or Cook syndrome.

■■■ NAIL PROFILE

The normal nail exhibits both transverse and longitudinal convex curvatures. The transverse curvature is more pronounced than the longitudinal one, and there are characteristic differences between finger- and toenails. There are considerable interindividual differences.

The nail may present a pathological curvature in either the longitudinal or the transverse direction, or in both. The nail may be overcurved, flat, or spoon-shaped.

The **parrot-beak nail (unguis inflexus)** is a peculiar, symmetrical overcurvature of the free margin of some fingernails simulating the beak of a parrot (Figure 2.37), but it may also develop when the bone of the terminal phalanx is shortened or the dorsal tuft supporting the nail bed is dislocated palmarwards.[42] It is a common finding in the acral type of scleroderma or after trauma with partial amputation of the terminal phalanx. However, this anomaly only develops when the nail bed is longer than the underlying bone and is thus pulled volarly around the tip of the bone. It is not seen in ter-

minal osteolysis due to tertiary hyperparathyroidism that develops during long-term hemodialysis; in contrast, an acquired brachyonychia develops in this condition (see above).

An inflexed nail is also seen in **pterygium inversum unguis** where the distal nail bed tissue adheres to the ventral surface of the nail plate, bending it down. It is frequently encountered after a trauma shortening the terminal phalanx, and is much less commonly seen in inflammatory diseases such as dermatomyositis.[43]

Hippocratic nails exhibit an exaggerated transverse and longitudinal curvature and often appear abnormally large[44] (Figure 2.38). They are part of a more complex abnormality: **finger clubbing** or **drumstick digit**. The distal phalanx is enlarged and round, and the nail is curved like the glass of a watch. The lunulae are abnormally large. The entire phalanx is commonly cyanotic. Initially, there is an increase in subungual connective tissue, with more fibroblasts. Later, a hyaline degeneration of the ground substance is seen. Finally, marked vascularization with increase in connective tissue and edema as well as an infiltrate composed of lymphocytes, plasma cells, and fibroblasts is seen. The nail plate becomes markedly hypertrophic. This condition

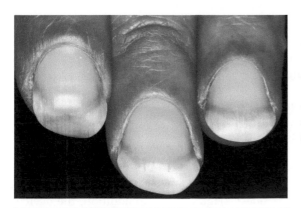

■ **FIGURE 2.37**

Parrot-beak nail.

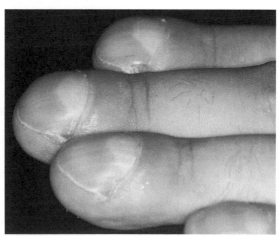

■ **FIGURE 2.38**

Finger clubbing.

is commonly seen in cor pulmonale and other cardiopulmonary diseases causing chronic hypoxemia. However, it may also be genetic, and a great number of other associated diseases have been described in the literature (Table 2.1). Recent research has shown that when platelet precursors fail to become fragmented into platelets within the pulmonary circulation, they are easily trapped in the peripheral vasculature, releasing platelet-derived growth factor (PDGF) and vascular endothelial growth factor (VEGF). These are promoters of vascularity and are thought to ultimately cause clubbing.

An increase in size of only one nail should raise the suspicion of a subungual tumor, which may be benign,[45] malignant, or metastatic.

Barrel-shaped **transverse overcurvature**, usually associated with oncholysis, is seen in acral **scleroderma**.

Transverse overcurvature, more pronounced on finger- than toenails, is a very characteristic sign of **scleronychia syndrome**,[46] which, when the nails become yellow, is known as **yellow nail syndrome**. The nails are thick, opaque, lusterless, and onycholytic. Because of the extremely slow growth rate, the cuticle disappears and there also develops a certain degree of separation of the eponychium from the undersurface of the proximal nail fold. The classical syndrome associates yellow, slowly growing nails with chronic bronchial infections, rhinosinusitis, and lymphedema.

In **pachyonychia congenita**, the nail plate is deformed in a horseshoe manner, covering a huge nail bed hyperkeratosis. The overcurvature increases slightly in the distal direction (Figure 2.39).

Overcurvature of the big toenails is common in **ingrown nails**, and it is a common observation that flat toenails virtually never develop this condition.

There are three types of transverse overcurvature of the big toenail: in **tile nails** (Figure 2.40), the overcurvature shows the same degree over its entire length, in **pincer nails** it increases distally (Figures 2.41 and 2.42), while in **plicated nails**,

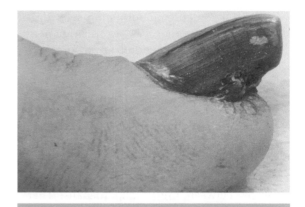

■ FIGURE 2.39

Pachyonychia congenita.

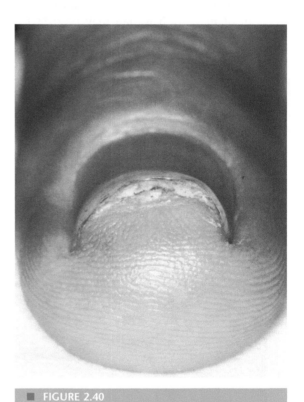

■ FIGURE 2.40

Transverse overcurvature in tile nail.

the nail plate shows a sharp bend on one or both sides[47] (Figure 2.43). In addition, the overcurvature may be seen only on one side of the nail as a so-called hemi-overcurvature.

■ TABLE 2.1

Possible causes of clubbing

IDIOPATHIC AND HEREDITARY DIGITAL CLUBBING

Congenital clubbing: familial, racial

Citrullinemia

ACQUIRED CLUBBING OF ALL DIGITS

Cardiopulmonary diseases (>80% of all cases of clubbing)

Congential heart disease

Congestive cardiac failure

Pulmonary artery malformations

Subacute bacterial endocarditis (Osler's disease)

Heart myxoma

Raynaud's disease

Maffucci syndrome

Bronchiectasis

Lung abscess

Lung cyst

Emphysema

Mucoviscidosis

Sarcoidosis

Infantile asthma

Chronic pneumonia

Pulmonary blastomycosis

Lung tuberculosis

Lung fibrosis

Hematological diseases

Polycythemia vera

Secondary polycythemia

Chronic methemoglobinemia

Poisoning with alcohol, arsenic, beryllium, mercury, phosphorus

Gastrointestinal diseases

Cancer of the esophagus, stomach, colon; leiomyosarcoma

Diseases of the small intestine

Chronic colonic diseases: amebiasis, Crohn's disease, colitis, ascariasis, schistosomiasis, whipworm (*Trichuris trichiura*)
    infection

Familiar polyposis

Gardner syndrome

Active chronic hepatitis

Hepatorenal syndrome

Purgative abuse

Possible causes of clubbing (*continued*)

Endocrine disorders

POEMS syndrome

Thyroid disease: pretibial myxedema, exophthalmos, finger clubbing (Diamond syndrome)

Thyroid cancer

Seipp–Lawrence syndrome

Miscellaneous diseases

AIDS

Hypervitaminosis A

Drug abuse: heroin, cannabis

Malnutrition, kwashiorkor

Syringomyelia

Lupus erythematosus

Professional: acro-osteolysis due to vinyl chloride

Unilateral clubbing

Aortal, subclavian, axillary, or ulnar artery aneurysm or stenosis

Ductus arteriosus

Arteriovenous fistula

Causalgia

Hemiplegia

Juvenile hyaline fibromatosis II

Pancoast tumor

Sarcoidosis

Shoulder subluxation

Unidigital clubbing

Tophaceous gout

Idiopathic

Local injury: whitlow, lymphangitis

Subungual epidermoid inclusions

Enchondroma

Osteoid osteoma

Varices of the arm

Takayasu's arteritis

Clubbing confined to upper or lower extremities

Hands: drug abuse

Feet: septic aortal graft

Transitory clubbing

Neonatal, due to reversal of the circulation after birth

Pseudoclubbing

Transverse and longitudinal overcurvature of the nail with normal Lovibond's angle: often due to subungual tumors

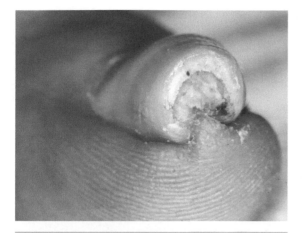

■ FIGURE 2.41
Acquired pincer nail.

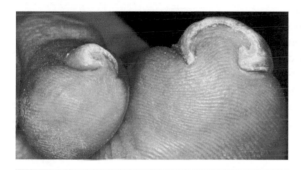

■ FIGURE 2.42
Congenital pincer nails.

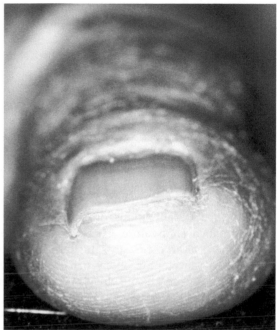

■ FIGURE 2.43
Plicated nail on both sides.

The most pronounced transverse overcurvature is seen in **pincer nails**. There are at least four different etiological groups of this condition: genetic, post-traumatic and due to foot deformation, during or after particular dermatoses, due to degenerative osteoarthritis of the distal interphalangeal finger joints with Heberden nodes, and submatrical tumors. The hereditary form of pincer nails commonly starts insidiously during the third or fourth decade of life with a distally pronounced transverse overcurvature of the hallux nail. The nail slowly deviates laterally. Very often, one or more of the lesser toes also develop transverse overcurvature; however, these nails always show a medial devi-

ation of their longitudinal axis. The symmetry of the toe involvement is striking. With time, the overcurvature increases, pinching the nail bed (unguis constringens), which thickens and develops a considerable subungual hyperkeratosis. In extreme cases, the free margin of the nail forms a complete tube (unguis convolutus). Although some patients complain of tenderness or even severe pain, most afflicted persons remain surprisingly asymptomatic. The mechanism of the distal overcurvature is evident when an X-ray film is taken: there are lateral osteophytes on both sides of the base of the terminal phalanx, with the medial one being considerably larger than the lateral one. They can usually be palpated as a step formation on the lateral aspect of the distal phalanx of the big toe. The osteophytes push the matrix horns apart, thus unbending the normally curved nail plate proximally, which in turn causes an overcurvature distally. Since the medial osteophyte is larger and in most cases formed like a hook that points distally, the medial matrix horn is pushed more forward deviating the longitudinal axis of the nail to the lateral side. Corresponding bony changes are also seen in the lesser toes.[48,49]

Pincer nails sometimes develop in the course of **psoriatic osteoarthropathy**, particularly when a secondary foot deformation or a psoriatic pachydermoperiostosis (acropachy) is seen. They do not progress to the degree that is often seen in the hereditary forms. The mechanism of development is probably similar.

Foot deformation and **trauma** may also lead to bone alterations of toes that translate into nail overcurvature. These changes are not symmetrical, in contrast to the hereditary form.

Slowly developing pincer nails of the fingers are typically seen in the elderly with **degenerative osteoarthritis** with Heberden nodes on their distal interphalangeal joints. We have seen an 82-year-old woman who developed a putrid long-standing paronychia with increasing overcurvature of this nail, which flattened spontaneously after successful treatment of her infection.

Tumors and other infiltrates bulging the matrix also cause an overcurvature. Depending on their location within the matrix, the overcurvature may be symmetrical or, when the tumour is located more laterally, hemi-overcurvature will develop. This is typically seen in subungual myxoid pseudocysts (Figure 2.44), usually in association with a violaceous discoloration of the area above the lesion.

Particularly in elderly persons, one or both edges of the nail may bend sharply, giving rise to a plicated nail. This abnormality is more frequent on toes than on fingers. Pressure on the nail from tight shoes may hurt and induce a hyperkeratosis in the lateral nail groove – onychophosis – which intensifies the pain.

Koilonychia (spoon nails) (Figure 2.45) and **platonychia (flat nails)** are just stages in the development of the same process. The surface slowly becomes concave and may finally look like a spoon. It has been suggested that

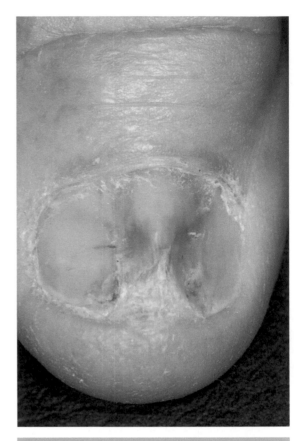

■ **FIGURE 2.44**

Subungual myxoid pseudocyst.

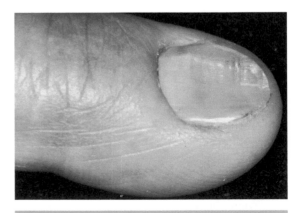

■ **FIGURE 2.45**

Koilonychia.

koilonychia is due to a disturbance of synchronized nail plate formation, with either the distal matrix or the nail bed growing faster than the proximal matrix. In most cases, this anomaly disappears spontaneously. Spoon nails are a physiological phenomenon in neonates. Many causes are listed in the literature, including iron deficiency, vitamin B_2 deficiency, trauma, avitaminosis C, and gastritis, and they have also been observed in patients with sprue, typhus, pellagra, Cushing's disease, or hyperthyroidism. In addition, there are idiopathic and hereditary cases; the latter may be associated with leukonychia.[50] Platonychia is also seen in trichothiodystrophy.

Longstanding mechanical strain to the pulp of the toes with gradual dislocation of the soft tissue over the tip of the digit also causes a spoon-like deformation of the nails known as **rickshaw nails**.

Solutions of salt and thioglycolate may also induce koilonychia.[51]

Onychogryposis (usually incorrectly spelled as onychogryphosis – *grypos* (Greek) means claw, *gryphos* is a prey bird) is a chronic condition with extreme ram's horn-like thickening of the nails, mainly toenails (Figure 2.46). It is predominantly observed in elderly and debilitated persons not able to care for themselves and for their nails. The nails are transformed into horn-like masses that may grow upwards and are often

bent. Their surface is irregular. There is no longer any attachment to the nail bed and the nail pocket is very short.[52] There is often an association with foot deformation. Some cases appear to be hereditary. Onychogryposis of finger nails may be due to chronic candidosis or even exposure to ionizing radiation.

■ ■ ■   **REFERENCES**

1. Baker H, Golding DN, Thompson M. The nail in psoriatic arthritis. Br J Dermatol 1964; 76: 569.
2. Eastmond CJ, Wright V. The nail dystrophy of psoriatic arthritis. Ann Rheum Dis 1979; 38: 226.
3. Piraccini BM, Fanti PA, Morelli R, Tosti A. Hallopeau's acrodermatitis continua of the nail apparatus: a clinical and pathological study of 20 patients. Acta Derma Venereol 1994; 74: 65–7.
4. Mahowald ML, Parrish RM. Severe osteolytic arthritis mutilans pustular psoriasis. Arch Dermatol 1982; 118: 434.
5. Cornelius CE, Shelley WB. Permanent anonychia due to lichen planus. Arch Dermatol 1967; 96; 434–5.
6. Pall A, Gupta RR, Gulati B, Goyal P. Twenty nail anonychia due to lichen planus. J Dermatol 2004; 31: 146–7.
7. Haneke E. Fungal infections of the nail. Semin Dermatol 1991; 10: 41–53.
8. Hashimoto H, Tsuda H, Takasaki Y. Digital ulcers/gangrene and immunoglobulin classes complement fixation antl dsDNA in systemic lupus erythematosus patients. J Rheumatol 1983; 10: 727–32.
9. Yang SG, Kim KH, Park KC. A case of systemic lupus erythematosus showing acute gangrenous change of fingertips. Br J Dermatol 1996; 134: 178–92.
10. Heller J. Lupus erythematodes der Nägel. Dermatol Z. 1906: 13: 613–15.
11. Tosti A, De Padova MP, Fanti P, Bonelli U, Taffurelli M. Unusual severe nail involvement in dermatomyositis. Cutis 1987; 40: 261–2.
12. Rowell NR. Acral pansclerotic morphea with intractable pain. In: Wilkinson DS, Mascaró JM, Orfanos C, eds. Case Collection Congressus Mundi Dermatologiae. Stuttgart: Schattauer, 1987: 178–80.
13. Schlesinger N, Katz M, Ingber A. Nail involvement in pemphigus vulgaris. Br J Dermatol 2002; 146: 836–9.
14. Leroy D, Lebrun J, Maillard V, et al. Pemphigus végétant à type clinique de dermatitis pustuleuse chronique de Hallopeau. Ann Dermatol Venereol 1982; 109: 549–55.
15. Török L, Husz S, Ocsai H, Krischner A, Kiss M. Pemphigus vegetans presenting as acrodermatitis continua suppurativa. Eur J Dermatol 2003; 13: 579–81.
16. Azulay RD. Brazilian pemphigus foliaceus. Int J Dermatol 192; 21: 122–4.
17. Tomita M, Tanei R, Hamada Y, Fujimura T, Katsuoka K. A case of localized pemphigoid with loss of toenails. Dermatology 2002; 204: 155
18. Bruge SM, Powell SM, Ryan TJ. Cicatricial pemphigoid with nail dystrophy. Clin Exp Dermatol 1985, 10: 472–5.

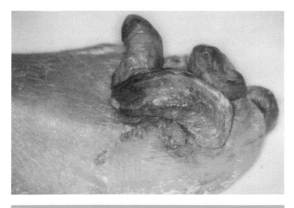

■   **FIGURE 2.46**

Onychogryposis.

19. McCuaig CC, Chan LS, Woodley DT, et al. Epidermolysis bullosa acquisita in childhood. Differentiation from hereditary epidermolysis bullosa. Arch Dermatol 1989; 125: 944–9.

20. Pal S, Haroon TS. Erythroderma: a clinico-etiologic study of 90 cases. Int J Dermatol. 1998; 37: 104–7.

21. Cholez C, Cuny JF, Pouaha J, et al. Nail abnormalities and scleroderma-like lesions on the face associated with systemic amyloidosis. Ann Dermatol Venereol 2005; 132: 252–4.

22. Guillaud V, Moulin G, Bonnefoy M, et al. Photo-onycholyse bulleuse au course d'une pseudoporphyrie des hémodialysés. Ann Dermatol Venereol 1990; 117: 723–5.

23. Scheinman LL, Helm KF, Fairley JA. Acral necrosis in a patient with chronic renal failure. Arch Dermatol 1991; 127: 247–52.

24. Kaur I, Chakrabati A, Dogra S, Rai R, Kumar B. Nail involvement in leprosy: a study of 300 patients. Int J Lepr Mycobact Dis 2003; 71: 320–7.

25. Leopold A, Wassilew SW. Hautveränderungen bei Syringomyelie. Z Hautkr 1988; 63: 494–6.

26. Haneke E. Hidrotic ectodermal dysplasias. In: R Happle, E Grosshans, eds. Pediatric Dermatology. Advances in Diagnosis and Treatment. Berlin: Springer-Verlag, 1987: 46.

27. Forni GL, Melevendi C, Jappelli S, Rasore-Quartino A. Dyskeratosis congenita: unusual presenting features within a kindred. Pediatr Hematol Oncol 1993; 10: 145–9.

28. Tang WY, Lee KC, Chow TC, Lo KK. Three Hong Kong Chinese cases of pretibial epidermolysis bullosa: a genodermatosis that can masquerade as an acquired inflammatory disease. Clin Exp Dermatol 1999; 24: 149–53.

29. Hintner H, Wolff K. Generalized atrophic benign epidermolysis bullosa. Arch Dermatol 1982; 118: 375.

30. Singalavanija S, Phuvichit B, Palungwachira P. Epidermolysis bullosa letalis (Herlitz disease): a case report. J Med Assoc Thai 1994; 77: 103–7.

31. Al Aboud K, Al Hawsawi K, Al Aboud D, Al Ghitami A. Kindler syndrome in a Saudi kindred. Clin Exp Dermatol 2002; 27: 673–6.

32. Happle R, Koch H, Lenz W. CHILD syndrome: congenital hemidysplasia with erythroderma and limb defects. Eur J Pediatr 1980; 134: 27.

33. Quinlan KE, Janiga JJ, Baran R, Lim HW. Transverse melanonychia secondary to total skin electron beam therapy. A report of 3 cases. J Am Acad Dermatol 2005; 53 S112–14.

34. Baran R, Juhlin L. Bone dependent nail formation. Br J Dermatol 1986; 114: 371–5.

35. Ronchese F. The racket thumbnail. Dermatologica 1973; 146: 199–202.

36. Alkiewicz J. Zur Klinik und Histologie der Anonychie. Arch Dermatol Syph 1938; 178: 234–9.

37. Nevin NC, Thomas PS, Eedy DJ, Shepherd C. Anonychia and absence/hypoplasia of distal phalanges (Cook's syndrome): report of a second family. J Med Genet 1995; 32: 638–41.

38. Sato U, Kitanaka S, Sekine T, et al. Functional characterization of *LMX1B* mutations associated with nail–patella syndrome. Paediatr Res 2005; 57: 783–8.

39. Baran R. Iso Kikuchi syndrome (C.O.I.F. syndrome). A report on 2 cases and a review of 44 cases in the literature. Ann Dermatol Venereol 1980; 107: 431–5.

40. Itin PH, Keseru B, Hauser V. Syndactyly/brachyphalangy and nail dysplasias as marker lesions for sclerosteosis. Dermatology 2001; 202: 259–60.

41. Burlina AB, Sherwood WG, Zacchello F. Partial biotinidase deficiency associated with Coffin–Siris syndrome. Eur J Pediatr 1990; 149: 628–9.

42. Pandya AN, Giele HP. Prevention of the parrot beak deformity in fingertip injuries. Hand Surg 2001; 6: 163–6.

43. Mello Filho A. Occurrence of pterygium inversum unguis in an adult population. Med Cutan Ibero Lat Am 1985; 13: 401–5.

44. Spicknall KE, Zirwas MJ, English JC. Clubbing: an update on diagnosis, differential diagnosis, pathophysiology, and clinical relevance. J Am Acad Dermatol 2005; 52: 1020–8.

45. Bukhari IA, Al-Mugharbel R. Subungual epidermoid inclusions. Saudi Med J 2004; 25: 522–3.

46. Samman PD, White WF. The yellow nail syndrome. Br J Dermatol 1964; 76: 153–7.

47. Hoffmann E. Doppelkantennägel. Zbl Haut-GeschlKr 1933; 47: 45.

48. Haneke E. Pincer nails (incurvated nail, unguis constringens, transverse overcurvature, trumpet nail, convoluted nail, and omega nail). In: Krull E, Baran R, Zook E, Haneke E. Nail Surgery: A Text and Atlas. New York: Lippincott Williams & Wilkins, 2001: 167–71.

49. Baran R, Haneke E, Richert B. Pincer nails: definition and surgical treatment. Dermatol Surg 2001; 27: 261–6.

50. Baran R, Achten G. Les associations congénitales de koïlonychie et de leuconychie totale. Arch Belg Dermatol 1969; 25: 13.

51. Hannuksela M, Hassi J. Hairdresser's hand. Derm Beruf Umwelt 1980; 28: 149–51.

52. Lubach D. Erbliche Onychogrypose. Hautarzt 1982; 33: 331.

Chapter 3

Subungual hyperkeratosis

Subungual hyperkeratosis is a common alteration and is seen in many conditions, particularly in chronic inflammatory diseases and chronic irritation of the nail bed. It is rarely specific, but may aid in a diagnosis in association with other signs. It often contains serum inclusions of variable size, inflammatory cells, and fungal elements. In this chapter, the lifting of the nail caused by hyperkeratosis of the distal nail bed will be discussed.

■■■ DERMATOLOGICAL DISEASES

Psoriasis often causes subungual hyperkeratosis, but its degree is extremely variable. The hyperkeratosis is usually loose and tends to break out, leaving residual onycholysis (Figure 3.1). There is a yellowish color shining through the nail. Its proximal margin typically has a reddish-brown colour (Figure 3.2). In fact, psoriatic distal nail bed hyperkeratosis is exactly the same as a salmon spot, but extending to the hyponychium. Extreme subungual hyperkeratosis (Figure 3.3) reminiscent of pachyonychia congenita is rare in psoriasis. Taking a piece, preferably the most proximal one, and submitting it for histopathological diagnosis can be very helpful, and often allows a definite diagnosis. In psoriasis, this hyperkeratosis contains large amounts of parakeratosis and often also Munro's microabscesses in different layers of the keratosis (Figure 3.4).

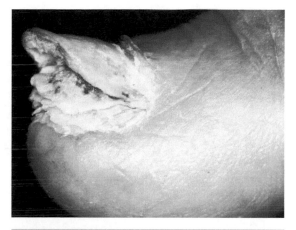

■ FIGURE 3.1
Psoriatic subungual hyperkeratosis lifting up the nail plate.

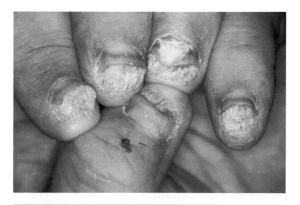

■ FIGURE 3.2
Psoriatic subungual hyperkeratosis involving all the digits. Reddish-brown color of the proximal margin.

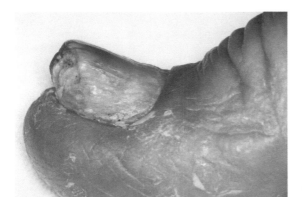

■ FIGURE 3.3

Psoriatic extreme subungual hyperkeratosis.

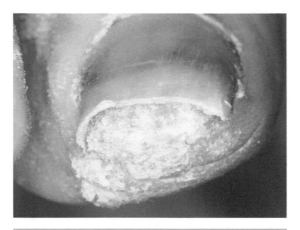

■ FIGURE 3.4

Psoriatic subungual hyperkeratosis with involvement of the tip of the digit.

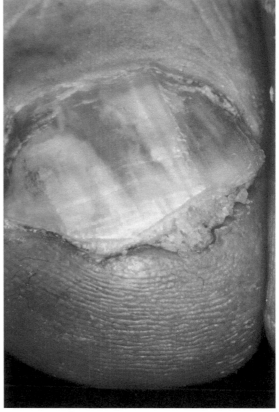

■ FIGURE 3.5

Distal–lateral subungual onychomycosis (DLSO) (*Trichophyton rubrum*).

This is a valuable histological feature for the differential diagnosis of psoriasis and onychomycosis, because some fungi may be seen even in psoriatic nails (see below).

Onychomycosis is the most frequent nail disease. **Distal subungual onychomycosis** often develops a reactive subungual hyperkeratosis (Figures 3.5–3.7), which, depending on the severity of the fungal infection, may reach the matrix. Histopathology usually demonstrates fungi, but neutrophils and dried serum inclusions are commonplace and may mimic nail

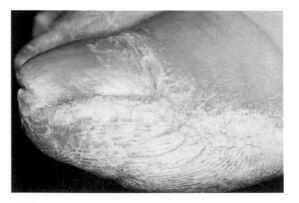

■ FIGURE 3.6

DLSO with hyperkeratosis of the pulp (*Trichophyton rubrum*).

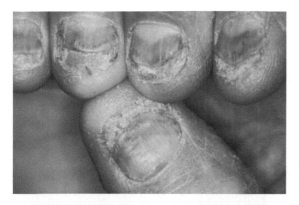

■ FIGURE 3.7

One-hand–two-foot tinea (*Trichophyton rubrum*).

psoriasis (see below). It has been found that the degree of subungual hyperkeratosis can be a predictive factor for a cure of onychomycosis or treatment failure.[1] Recently, a case of onychomycosis with massive subungual hyperkeratosis harboring the booklouse *Liposcelis* has been described.[2]

An onychomycosis that was assumed to be due to *Malassezia furfur* presented with subungual hyperkeratosis and subsequent onycholysis.[3]

Some chronic cases of distal subungual onychomycosis may cause very pronounced subungual hyperkeratosis and sometimes also onychauxis (Figure 3.8).

Contact **allergic eczema** (Figure 3.9) of the fingertips due to sensitization to cyanoacrylate adhesive has been observed to induce prominent nail bed hyperkeratosis in addition to onycholysis and nail dystrophy.[4] Cement workers are prone to present subungual hyperkeratosis (Figure 3.10a) as well as chemical users (Figure 3.10b) and particularly epoxy resin (Figure 3.10c).

Crusted scabies may present with hyperkeratotic psoriasis-like accumulations of scales under the nails (Figure 3.11). This dystrophy may be the most important marker of the persistence of this type of infestation.

Pityriasis rubra pilaris (see Chapter 1, Figure 1.33) involving the nails usually starts as hyperkeratosis of the distal nail bed. Distal

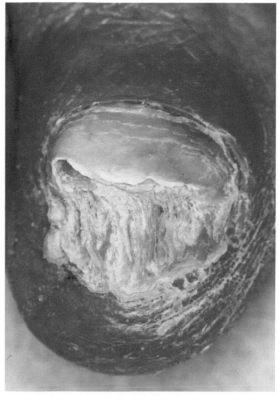

■ FIGURE 3.8

DLSO with extreme hyperkeratosis (*Trichophyton rubrum*).

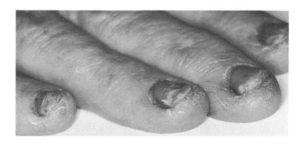

■ FIGURE 3.9

Contact dermatitis: subungual hyperkeratosis due to acrylic nails.

yellow–brown discoloration, subungual hyperkeratosis, nail plate thickening, and splinter hemorrhages indicate a diagnosis of adult (type 1) pityriasis rubra pilaris rather than psoriasis,

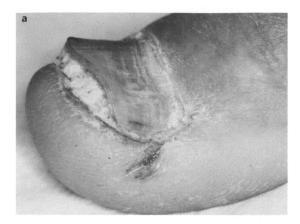

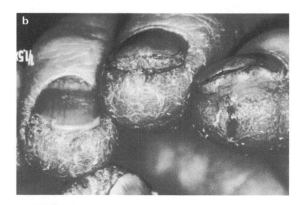

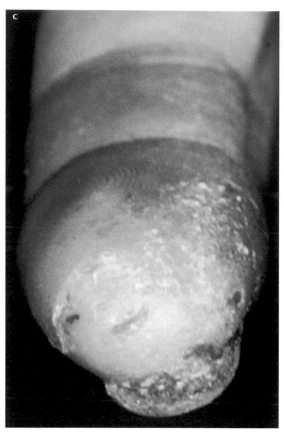

■ **FIGURE 3.10**

Contact dermatitis: (a) in a cement worker; (b) due to chemicals; (c) due to epoxy resin. (Part (c) courtesy of JF Fowler, USA.)

which is rather characterized by onycholysis (particularly marginal), salmon patches, small pits, and larger indentations of the nail plate. The nail changes of pityriasis rubra pilaris were thought to be reactive rather than specific, as similar changes were seen in patients with long-standing erythroderma due to Sézary syndrome[5] (Figure 3.12).

Common warts (Figures 3.13 and 3.14) when localized on the hyponychium cause considerable hyperkeratosis thickening the nail plate. They may even erode the bone and cause pain.[6] We have seen relatively flat warts form-ing a rim around the hyponychium of both big toenails, which were swollen after a bath and took on a white color due to hydration. Histopathology showed only a slight epidermal acanthosis with a few koilocytes and coarse ker-atohyaline granules, but in situ hybridization for human papilloma virus (HPV) type 3 was positive.

Subungual **keratoacanthoma** (Figure 3.15) often starts as a tender wart-like subungual hyperkeratosis that soon becomes characteristi-cally painful.[7] Upon pressure, the horn plug fill-ing the central crater can sometimes be partially

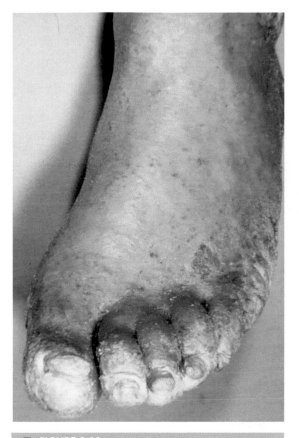

FIGURE 3.11

Crusted scabies.

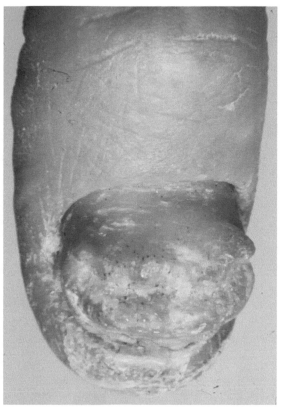

FIGURE 3.13

Subungual warts.

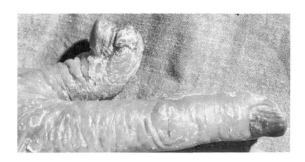

FIGURE 3.12

Sézary syndrome.

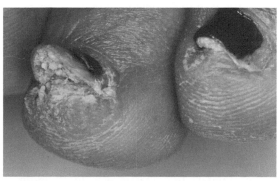

FIGURE 3.14

Subungual warts lifting up the nail plate.

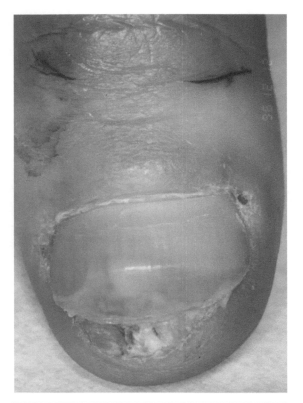

■ FIGURE 3.15

Keratoacanthoma.

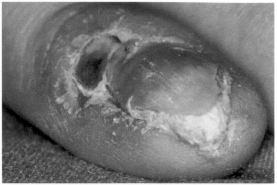

■ FIGURE 3.16

Discoid lupus erythematosus. (Courtesy of B Richert, Belgium.)

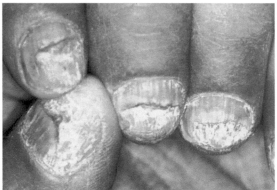

■ FIGURE 3.17

Subungual hyperkeratosis in lichen planus.

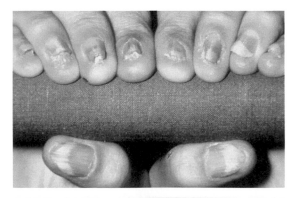

■ FIGURE 3.18

Nonscarring recessive epidermolysis bullosa. (Courtesy of I Anton-Lamprecht, Germany.)

expressed. Multiple lesions have been observed.[8] A radiograph may demonstrate erosion of the tip of the terminal phalangeal bone.

Unusually severe distal subungual hyperkeratosis has been described in a case of chronic discoid **lupus erythematosus** (Figure 3.16) that later evolved into systemic lupus erythematosus.[9]

Lichen planus may present with subungual hyperkeratosis alone or in combination with onycholysis (Figure 3.17).

Epidermolysis bullosa acquisita, an autoimmune dermatosis with autoantibodies against collagen type VII, may rarely lead to subungual hyperkeratosis.[10] In epidermolysis bullosa (dystrophic, localized, or generalized), the nails may be thick (Figure 3.18).

■ ■ ■ SYSTEMIC CONDITIONS

Subungual hyperkeratosis is commonly seen in the nail changes induced by **β-blockers**. Together with brown discoloration, it has also been seen in high-dose **clofazimine** treatment for lepromatous leprosy.[11]

Subungual hyperkeratosis is a typical feature of **acrokeratosis paraneoplastica of Bazex**[12] (Figure 3.19) (see Chapter 1).

It may also occur in the different forms of acropachy.

■ ■ ■ GENETIC DISEASES

Pachyonychia congenita (PC) is the hereditary disease with the most pronounced subungual hyperkeratosis (Figure 3.20). Four types are known,[13] two of which are defined as

defects in the genes for the keratin pairs 6a/16 (Jadassohn–Lewandowski type or type 1) and 6b/17 (Jackson–Lawler type or type 2). To date, many different missense mutations have been found, but the clinical expression is almost always the same. These keratins are normally expressed in the nail bed, but not or much less in the matrix; this is the reason why an almost normal nail plate covers a huge hyperkeratosis of the nail bed. The nail plate overlies the keratosis in a horseshoe-like manner. PC is usually inherited as an autosomal dominant trait, although an autosomal recessive case has been described.

Type 1 is most common with approximately 55% of all PC cases. All nails become yellowish-brown to dirty greenish-gray shortly after birth

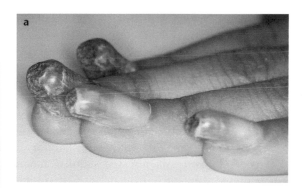

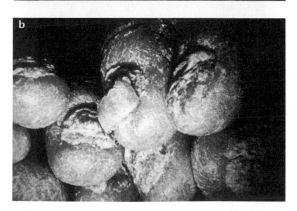

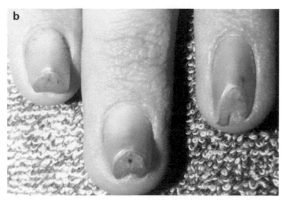

■ FIGURE 3.19 (a,b)
Acrokeratosis paraneoplastica.

■ FIGURE 3.20 (a,b)
Pachyonychia congenita. (Part (b) courtesy of F Daniel, France.)

and develop a huge subungual hyperkeratosis elevating the nail plate from the nail bed. Other symptoms of the syndrome are blistering and patchy hyperkeratoses of the soles of the feet and palms of the hands, follicular hyperkeratoses, and oral leukokeratosis. However, exclusive nail involvement is not rare. Late-onset type 1 PC has repeatedly been described.[14]

In type 2 (approximately 25% of PC cases), there are in addition multiple steatocystomas, often beginning during childhood, plus bullae of palms and soles, palmar and plantar hyperhidrosis, and natal or neonatal teeth. Eruptive vellus hair cysts and epidermoid cysts have also been observed.

Type 3 (about 12% of patients) has the symptoms of types 1 and 2 plus angular cheilosis, corneal dyskeratosis, and cataracts.

Type 4 (comprising about 7% of cases) has laryngeal lesions with hoarseness, hair abnomalies, and mental retardation in addition.

However, the classification is not always unequivocal, mixed-type cases have been described, and PC without the classical keratin gene mutations may occur.[15]

A peculiar form of PC has been described in which the nail changes tended to decrease with age. There was also moderate palmoplantar hyperkeratosis. All affected family members exhibited a characteristic pattern of cutaneous hyperpigmentation resembling macular amyloidosis around the neck and waist, but conferring a dappled appearance to the axillae, popliteal fossae, thighs, buttocks, and lower aspect of the abdomen. With advancing age, the pigmentation faded. Histological and ultrastructural examination of the hyperpigmented skin revealed pigmentary incontinence and deposition of amyloid within the papillary dermis. These features appear to constitute a distinct variant of PC.

A syndrome characterized by PC-like nail dystrophy, woolly hair, premature loss of teeth, acral hyperkeratosis, and facial abnormalities has been recently described in a Dutch kindred.[16]

It has been found through connexin 30 gene (*GJB6*) sequencing that PC-like nail changes may also be found in the Clouston type of tricho-onychotic ectodermal dysplasia.[17]

Subungual hyperkeratosis may be very marked in **dyskeratosis follicularis of Darier** (Figure 3.21). It is usually cuneiform and seen in association with longitudinal white and reddish lines that commonly end in V-shaped notches of the nail's free margin.[18] It is noteworthy that nail involvement may occur without other manifestations of Darier's disease.[19]

An **odonto-onychotic hypohidrotic ectodermal dysplasia** with onycholysis and subungual hyperkeratosis, hypoplastic enamel of the the teeth, and hypohidrosis that was inherited as an autosomal dominant trait was described by Witkop et al.[20]

■ ■ ■   MECHANICAL AND PHYSICAL CAUSES

Artificial nails of moderate length exert a lever action and have an impact on the nail attachment of the most distal nail bed, causing subungual hyperkeratosis; very long artificial

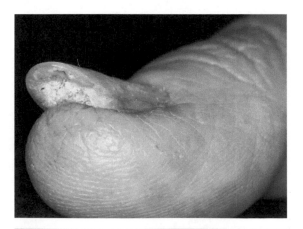

■   FIGURE 3.21

Darier's disease.

nails soon disrupt this attachment, leading to onycholysis.

Distal subungual hyperkeratosis has also been seen in a semiprofessional sailor due to intense strain on the free margin of the nails from grasping the sail tissue. Similar mechanically induced subungual hyperkeratoses are also seen in other professions and sports.

Wart and callus-resembling hyperkeratoses on both tips of the index fingers in close proximity to the hyponychium have been described under the term 'slot machine' finger, in a young man who used to play at a slot machine for approximately 7 hours each day.[21]

Keratosis cristarum is a peculiar type of distal nail bed hyperkeratosis that is associated with slight longitudinal ridge-like elevations of the nail plate – although without thickening of the nail plate at these sites (Figure 3.22). It slowly extends proximally, leading to distal onycholysis. Quite commonly, longitudinal red stripes are seen. The nature of keratosis cristarum is not yet clear.[22]

Another lesion of unclear etiology and pathogenesis is **localized multinucleate distal subungual keratosis**. This is seen under the nail plate and originates from an onychopapilloma, probably of the distal nail bed.[23] It may be associated with longitudinal erythronychia (see Chapter 6).

Pincer nails characteristically develop a subungual hyperkeratosis, the thickness of which is greatest where the overcurvature of the nail is most pronounced. Its ridged pattern is easily seen when the nail is avulsed. Serum inclusion are seen in a columnar arrangement in histological sections.[24]

Repeated minor trauma is the cause of **onychophosis** (Figure 3.23), a condition characterized by the development of painful calluses in the lateral nail grooves.

Repeated trauma is also the cause of **subungual corn (onychoclavus, heloma subunguale)**[25] (Figure 3.24). This is usually localized in the hyponychium or distal nail bed. Cutting the overlying nail plate away will make the lesion visible and also relieve the pain, as the pressure will be diminished.

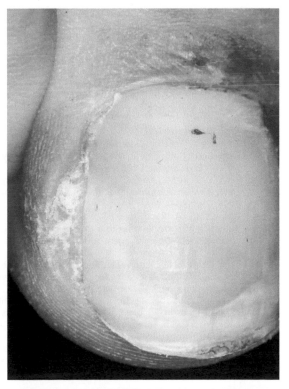

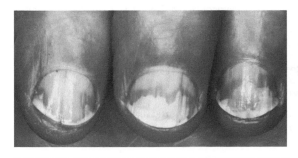

■ FIGURE 3.22

Keratosis cristarum. (Courtesy of C Beylot, France.)

■ FIGURE 3.23

Onychophosis.

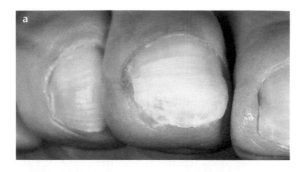

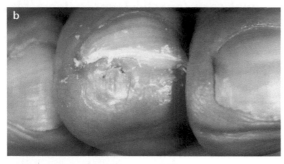

■ FIGURE 3.24 (a,b)

Onychoclavus. (Courtesy of S Goettmann-Bonvallot).

■■■ REFERENCES

1. Sommer S, Sheehan-Dare RA, Goodfield MJ, Evans EG. Prediction of outcome in the treatment of onychomycosis. Clin Exp Dermatol 2003; 28: 425–8.
2. Lin YC, Chan ML, Ko CW, Hsieh MY. Nail infestation by *Liposcelis bostrychophila* Badonnel. Clin Exp Dermatol 2004; 29: 620–1.
3. Chowdhary A, Randhawa HS, Sharma S, Brandt ME, Kumar S. *Malassezia furfur* in a case of onychomycosis: colonizer or etiologic agent? Med Mycol 2005; 43: 87–90.
4. Guin JD, Baas K, Nelson-Adesokan P. Contact sensitization to cyanoacrylate adhesive as a cause of severe onychodystrophy. Int J Dermatol 1998; 37: 31–6.
5. Sonnex TS, Dawber RP, Zachary CB, Millard PR, Griffiths AD. The nails in adult type 1 pityriasis rubra pilaris. A comparison with Sézary syndrome and psoriasis. J Am Acad Dermatol 1986; 15: 956–60.
6. Plewig G, Christophers E, Braun-Falco O. Mutilierende subunguale Warzen: Abheilung durch Methotrexat. Hautarzt 1973; 24: 338–41.
7. Baran R, Goettmann S. Distal digital keratoacanthoma. A report of 12 cases and a review of the literature. Br J Dermatol 1998; 139: 512–15.
8. Haneke E. Multiple subungual keratoacanthomas. Zbl Haut-GeschlKr 1991; 159: 337–8.
9. Richert B, André J, Bourguignon R, de la Brassinne M. Hyperkeratotic nail discoid lupus erythematosus evolving towards systemic lupus erythematosus: therapeutic difficulties. J Eur Acad Dermatol Venereol 2004; 18: 728–30.
10. McCuaig CC, Chan LS, Woodley DT, et al. Epidermolysis bullosa acquisita in childhood. Differentiation from hereditary epidermolysis bullosa. Arch Dermatol 1989; 125: 944–9.
11. Dixit VB, Chaudhary SD, Jain VK. Clofazimine induced nail changes. Int J Leprosy 1989; 61: 476–8.
12. Bolognia JL, Brewer YP, Cooper DL. Bazex syndrome (acrokeratosis paraneoplastica). An analytic review. Medicine (Baltimore) 1991; 70: 269–80.
13. Feinstein A, Friedman J, Schewach-Millet M. Pachyonychia congenita. J Am Acad Dermatol 1988; 19: 705–11.
14. Mouaci-Midoun N, Cambiaghi S, Abimelec P. Pachyonychia congenita tarda. J Am Acad Dermatol 1996; 35: 334–5.
15. van Steensel MA, Smith FJ, Steijlen PM. A new type of pachyonychia congenita. Eur J Dermatol 2001; 11: 188–90.
16. van Steensel MA, Koedam MI, Swinkels OQ, Rietveld F, Steijlen PM. Woolly hair, premature loss of teeth, nail dystrophy, acral hyperkeratosis and facial abnormalities: possible new syndrome in a Dutch kindred. Br J Dermatol 2001; 145: 157–61.
17. van Steensel MA, Jonkman MF, van Geel M, et al. Clouston syndrome can mimic pachyonychia congenita. J Invest Dermatol 2003; 121: 1035–8.
18. Burge SM, Wilkinson JD. Darier–White disease: a review of the clinical features of 163 patients. J Am Acad Dermatol 1992; 27: 40–50.
19. Bingham EA, Burrow D. Darier's disease. Br J Dermatol 1984; 111(Suppl 26): 88–9.
20. Witkop CJ Jr, Brearley LJ, Gentry WC Jr. Hypoplastic enamel, onycholysis, and hypohidrosis inherited as an autosomal dominant trait. A review of ectodermal dysplasia syndromes. Oral Surg Oral Med Oral Pathol. 1975; 39: 71–86.
21. Chaudhry SI, McGibbon D. 'Slot machine' finger: an occupational dermatosis? Clin Exp Dermatol 2005; 30: 90–1.
22. Alkiewicz J, Pfister R. Atlas der Nagelkrankheiten. Stuttgart: Schattauer, 1976: 118.
23. Baran R, Perrin C. Localized multinucleate distal subungual keratosis. Br J Dermatol 1995; 133: 77–82.
24. Haneke E. Etiopathogénie et traitement de l'hypercourbure transversale de l'ongle du gros orteil. J Méd Esth Chir Dermatol 1992; 19: 123–7.
25. Gilchrist AK. Common foot problems in the elderly. Geriatrics 1979; 34: 67–70.

Chapter 4

Onycholysis

Separation of the nail plate from the distal portion of the nail is commonly called **onycholysis**, whereas separation from the matrix and proximal nail bed is called **onychomadesis**. Onycholysis is a common phenomenon, and occurs in almost all patients with subungual hyperkeratosis (Figure 4.1). This latter condition will therefore not be discussed any further here, although distinction of onycholysis with and without subungual hyperkeratosis is often somewhat arbitrary. In many cases, there is a continuum of onycholysis with and without subungual hyperkeratosis. The most common causes of onycholysis are acute and chronic inflammation, parakeratosis, and trauma[1] (Table 4.1). As most cases of onycholysis start from the hyponychium and extend proximally, there is no primary matrix involvement. Psoriasis is an exception, as an oil spot may turn into onycholysis when it reaches the hyponychium (Figure 4.2).

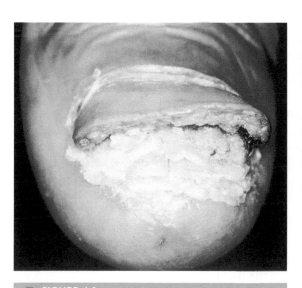

■ FIGURE 4.1

Psoriatic onycholysis associated with subungual hyperkeratosis.

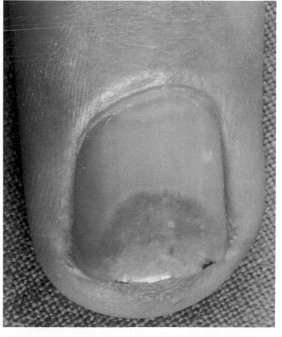

■ FIGURE 4.2

Oily spot in the distal nail bed.

■ TABLE 4.1
Causes of onycholysis

IDIOPATHIC

In women

Leuko-onycholysis paradentotica of Schuppli

LOCAL

Trauma: accidental, self-inflicted, occupational

Tumors of the nail bed

Foreign body

Infection: viral, bacterial, fungal

Chemical: prolonged water contact, alkali, detergents, bleach, organic solvents, nail polish removers, gasoline,
concentrated salt and sugar solution

Cosmetics: formaldehyde, false nails, depilatory products, nickel in metal pellets of nail varnish

DERMATOSES

Psoriasis, Reiter's disease, vesicular and bullous diseases, lichen planus, alopecia areata, eczema, multicentric
reticulohistocytosis, actinic reticuloid

SYSTEMIC

Pregnancy, iron-deficiency anemia, lung carcinoma, circulatory, lupus erythematosus, hypothyroidism, thyrotoxicosis,
syphilis, yellow nail syndrome

DRUGS

Cytotoxic drugs: bleomycin, docetaxel, doxorubicin, icodextrin, mitoxantrone, 5-fluorouracil (systemic and topical),
paclitaxel, retinoids

Photo-onycholysis: tetracyclines (particularly demeclocycline, and doxycycline, but also minocycline),
fluoroquinolones, photochemotherapy with psoralens, thiazide diuretics, flumequine, quinine, oral contraceptives,
indomethacin, captopril, trypaflavin, chlorpromazine, chloramphenicol, cephaloridine, icodextrin, allopurinol,
cloxacillin, clorazepate dipotassium

When the nail loses its adhesion to the nail bed, it loses its transparency and becomes yellowish. Irregularities of the nail plate surface hint at an additional matrix pathology.

■ ■ ■ DERMATOLOGICAL DISEASES

Distal onycholysis is one of the very characteristic signs of nail **psoriasis**. In contrast to the epidermis, in the nail, the irritation caused by the psoriatic inflammation will lead not only to marked parakeratosis, but also to the formation of a patchy granular layer. Loss of the nail plate–nail bed attachment is the consequence.[2,3] However, the cause of onycholysis is not always obvious, as various diseases may induce clinically similar pictures. It is said that psoriatic onycholysis can commonly be differentiated from mycotic onycholysis and other forms by its proximal reddish-brown margin (Figure 4.3). This corresponds to the active psoriatic lesion, and is identical to the salmon spot that is seen in the nail bed.

Distal subungual onychomycosis often causes primary onycholysis, almost without subungual hyperkeratosis (Figure 4.4). It is due to

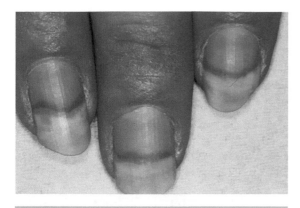

■ FIGURE 4.3

Psoriatic onycholysis with a proximal reddish-brown margin.

the formation of an abnormal granular layer in the nail bed. Dermatophytes may be cultured from otherwise normal looking onycholysis of the big toenail.[4]

Areas of onycholysis in the matrix and/or nail bed without connection to the pulp of the digit develop in **proximal subungual onychomycosis**. They stand out by their grayish-white color and loss of transparency[5] (Figure 4.5).

Primary 'idiopathic' onycholysis and secondary mycotic colonization or even infection preventing its healing is called **mycotic onycholysis**[5] (Figures 4.6 and 4.7).

Fingertip **eczema** of different types may cause subungual hyperkeratosis and/or onycholysis.[6, 7]

A characteristic picture is the **tulip finger**, with chronic chapping of the finger tips, fissures, and onycholysis. Other causes, such as **acrylates**

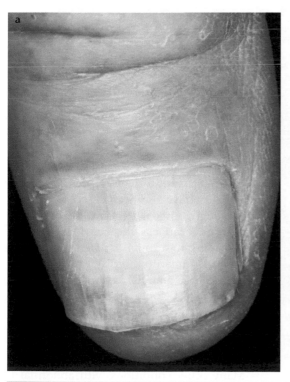
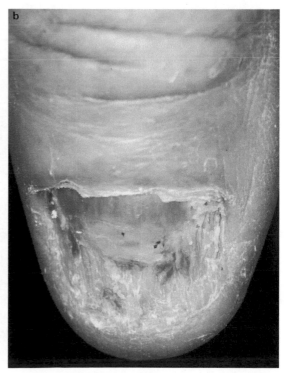

■ FIGURE 4.4

(a) Mycotic onycholysis. (b) In the same patient, the nail bed after section of the loose area.

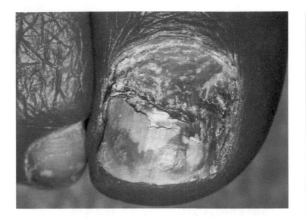

■ FIGURE 4.5

Proximal subungual onychomycosis with destruction of the proximal nail keratin. (Courtesy of DT Robert, UK.)

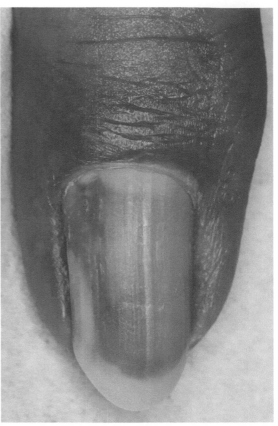

■ FIGURE 4.7

Secondary mycotic lateral onycholysis.

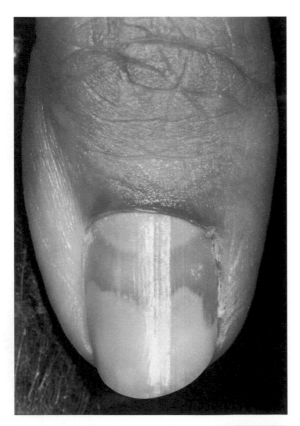

■ FIGURE 4.6

Secondary mycotic distal onycholysis.

(Figure 4.8) and formaldehyde nail hardener (Figure 4.9) have also been described.[8]

Although ungual **lichen planus** (Figure 4.10) usually attacks the proximal nail matrix first, leading to a rough striated surface, it may also affect primarily the distal nail bed. It typically induces a granular layer, and consequently onycholysis developing through nail bed hyperkeratosis has also been observed. Very rarely, **alopecia areata** may present with onycholysis, which disappears when the scalp condition improves (Figure 4.11).

Many other conditions with abnormal keratinization of the nail bed, including nail bed hyperkeratosis, also exhibit onycholysis. This is

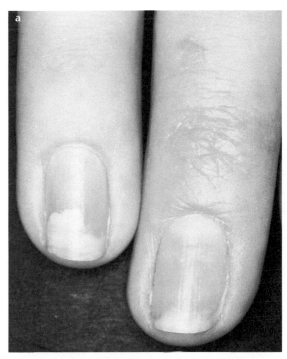

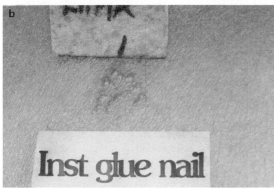

(a) Onycholysis due to cyanoacrylate. (Courtesy of L Kanerva, Finland.) (b) Positive test to the glue.

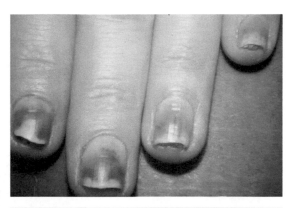

■ FIGURE 4.9

Subungual hyperkeratosis associated with hemorrhage, due to formaldehyde.

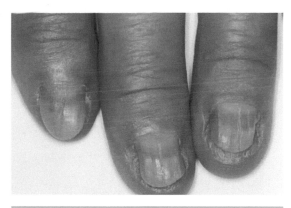

■ FIGURE 4.10

Lichen planus onycholysis (involvement of the nail bed).

seen in **dyskeratosis follicularis of Darier**, often in a V-shaped form.

Proximal onycholysis (onychomadesis), with or without ensuing nail shedding, occurs after severe exudative inflammation with blister formation: in **erythema multiforme, Stevens–Johnson syndrome**, and **Lyell syndrome** (Figure 4.12), but rarely also in **psoriasis** (Figure 4.13). **Acute subungual felon** also causes onychomadesis.

Scars of the distal nail bed usually result in circumscribed areas of onycholysis, as do **subungual tumors** in a distal location, particularly subungual exostoses. When Bowen's disease affects larger areas of the nail bed, the plate loses its attachment to the nail bed in this area. Onycholysis has also been observed after spontaneous regression of a subungual keratoacanthoma.[9]

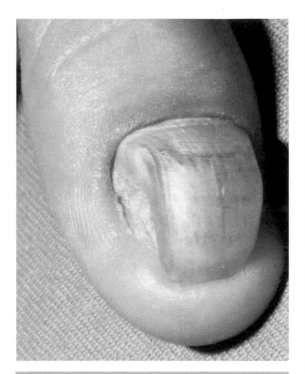

■ FIGURE 4.11

Onycholysis in alopecia areata.

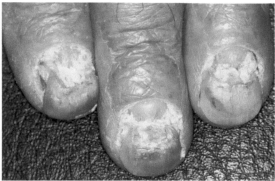

■ FIGURE 4.13

Psoriatic onychomadesis.

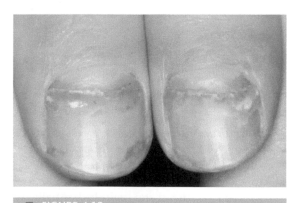

■ FIGURE 4.12

Onychomadesis in Lyell syndrome.

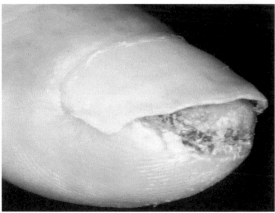

■ FIGURE 4.14

Onycholysis in secondary syphilis.

Secondary syphilis (Figure 4.14) may produce onycholysis. Another mechanism of onycholysis is the development of **granulation tissue** (Figure 4.15). In ingrown toenails, this may develop when a nail spicule has pierced the epidermis of the lateral nail groove. It may enlarge and spread under the nail plate, detaching it from the nail bed. However, this is also seen as an adverse effect of treatment with topical and systemic retinoids,[10] as well as with protease inhibitors, and different epidermal growth factor receptor (EGFR) inhibitors.[11]

■■■ SYSTEMIC CONDITIONS

When systemic diseases or drugs taken orally are the cause of onycholysis, it is usual for all finger-

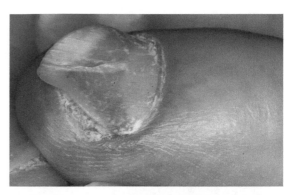

■ FIGURE 4.16
Iron-deficiency onycholysis associated with koilonychia.

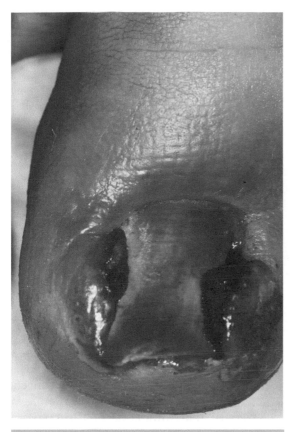

■ FIGURE 4.15
Granulation tissue associated with onycholysis due to an ingrowing toenail.

nails and to a lesser degree also the toenails to be involved according to their growth rate. Grossly asymmetrical involvement suggests a local cause.

Reiter's disease can cause severe onycholysis, which in one case of HIV infection cleared after infliximab therapy.[12]

Iron deficiency has long been known to cause not only spoon nails, but also onycholysis.[13]

Onycholysis is a typical feature of the **yellow nail syndrome** (Figure 4.16), which shows very slowly growing but thick nails, loss of the cuticle and the attachment to the undersurface of the proximal nail fold, transverse overcurvature, and a yellowish discoloration that may take on a brownish or greenish tinge.[14] The onycholysis

may progress toward the matrix and cause nail shedding. This syndrome has been long known in under the term of **scleronychia syndrome**, but the yellow color is not mandatory.[15]

Acrokeratosis paraneoplastica of Bazex usually causes distal onycholysis, but may sometimes cause onychomadesis[16,17] (Figure 4.17) – this is apparently a sign of an acute onset

Onycholysis is the most common nail symptom in **systemic lupus erythematosus (SLE)**[18] (Figure 4.18).

Other systemic causes may be severe **general diseases, peripheral arterial disease**, and **hyperthyroidism**. A particular syndrome of

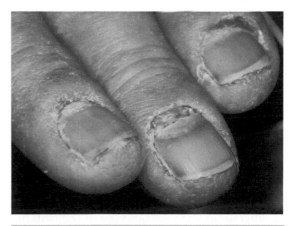

■ FIGURE 4.17
Acrokeratosis paraneoplastica.

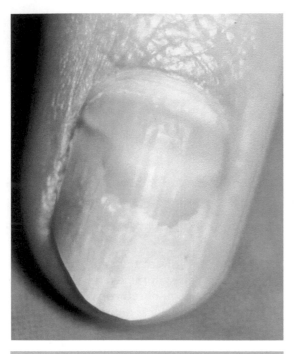

■ FIGURE 4.18

Onycholysis in systemic lupus erythematosus. (Courtesy of S Goettmann-Bonvallot, France.)

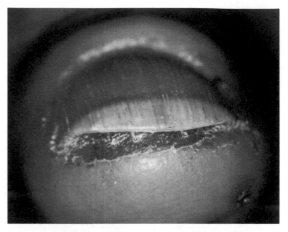

■ FIGURE 4.19

Onycholysis due to cytotoxic drugs.

thyrotoxicosis is characterized by exophthalmos, pretibial myxedema, acropachy, hippocratic nails, and onycholysis.

Drugs may cause onycholysis through an inflammatory mechanism, as seen during treatment with β-blockers, particularly those of the first generation.[19] Many more agents have been implicated in onycholysis (Figure 4.19), but their mechanism of action is often not known. Taxanes are known to cause onycholysis and a particular kind of subungual hemorrhagic abscess,[20–23] and some of these drugs may also cause photo-onycholysis. Docetaxel is probably among those with the most frequent nail side-effects, particularly onycholysis, which frequently limits its cumulative dose.[24–28] About 40% of docetaxel-treated patients develop painful onycholysis. Interestingly, these nail alterations were not observed in the nails on the right hand in a patient with a complete peripheral palsy of the right arm, whereas the nails of the other three extremities were affected.[22] It was postulated that an inflammatory process maintained by postganglionic sympathetic terminals and nociceptive C-fiber afferents was responsible, and improvement of the nail lesions was achieved following cyclooxygenase-2 inhibitor treatment. Taxane-induced onycholysis may progress to nail loss, but it has been suggested that withdrawal of paclitaxel is not necessary, as the nails may regrow normally despite continuation of treatment. Other cytotoxic agents may also cause onycholysis.[25,26] Mitoxantrone, a derivative of doxorubicin, has also been reported to induce onycholysis,[29–32] sometimes in association with a yellowish discoloration, subungual hemorrhage and abscess formation, pyogenic granuloma, and paronychia.[33] Etretinate may make one prone to onycholysis or onychomadesis (Figure 4.20). Pseudoporphyria (Figure 4.21) may result from a variety of drugs.

Photo-onycholysis after ingestion of photosensitizing drugs is a rare event. Most often, tetracyclines, particularly doxycycline,[34] are the cause, but other drugs (e.g. fluoroquinolones), photochemotherapy with psoralens (Figure 4.22), and even fruits containing photosensitizing ingredients such as figs, may cause photo-onycholysis. Recently, more drugs have

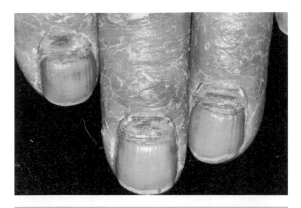

■ FIGURE 4.20

Onychomadesis due to etretinate in a psoriatic patient.

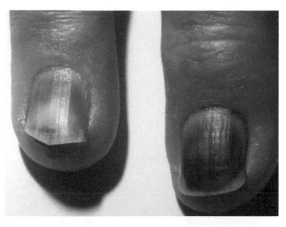

■ FIGURE 4.21

Pseudoporphyria with onycholysis and subungual hemorrhage. (Courtesy of JL Levy, France.)

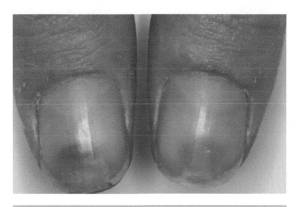

■ FIGURE 4.22

Photo-onycholysis (PUVA) therapy.

been added to the list of photo-onycholysis-inducing substances, for example sparfloxacin. Photo-onycholysis induced by paclitaxel and trastuzumab in association with aberrations of porphyrin metabolism has recently been described.

Some severe general diseases such as **scarlet fever, sepsis, pneumonia, hepatitis**, and **influenza**, have been blamed for onychomadesis. Recurrent forms have been described.

■■■ GENETIC DISEASES

Distal onycholysis was seen in an **ectodermal dysplasia** family over four generations with Marie–Unna-type hypotrichosis. Congenital partial onycholysis associated with thick and hard nails has been reported in some families[35] (Figure 4.23).

A purely **tricho-onychotic ectodermal dysplasia** characterized by hypotrichosis and onycholysis and by short, thickened, overcurved nails without cuticle has been described as a probable new mutation.

A family with an **autosomal recessive nail dysplasia** presenting with onycholysis of the fingers and anonychia of the toes in six generations has been described from Pakistan.

Onycholysis subsequent to subungual hemorrhages has been observed in **hyper-homocysteinemia** due to a defect in the gene for tetrahydrofolate reductase. Systemic administration of folic acid controlled the hyper-homocysteinemia and the cutaneous lesions, including the onycholysis.

■■■ MECHANICAL AND PHYSICAL CAUSES

Onycholysis semilunaris is probably the most common form. Most patients are female,

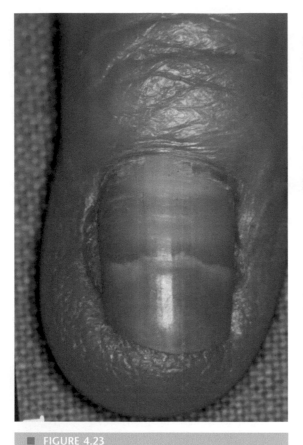

Hereditary partial onycholysis with sleronychia.

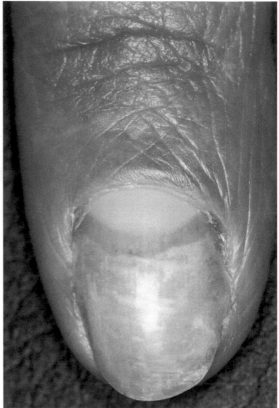

Secondary onycholysis (wet work).

and although they usually claim not to overdo manicure and avoid using sharp instruments, etc., this condition is generally accepted as being self-inflicted. The term onycholysis semilunaris explains the common half-moon-shaped area of onycholysis. The enlarged 'free nail' area is yellowish and there is no subungual hyperkeratosis (Figure 4.24). Dirt and microorganisms may be trapped under the free nail margin, inciting a vicious circle of overzealous cleaning of the space under the nail and exacerbation of the condition.

Onycholysis is a frequent consequence of long normal (Figure 4.25) or **artificial nails**, which exert a lever action overcoming the attachment forces of the nail bed with the nail plate. Again, the enlarged space under the normal nail is susceptible to secondary colonization with saprophytes and facultative and obligatory pathogens, worsening the onycholysis.

Occupational traumatic abnormalities in the nail region include major trauma (Figure 4.26), repeated microtrauma (Figure 4.27), and foreign body injury (Figure 4.28). Occupational onycholysis is most frequently due to chemical irritants or sensitizers. Long-term action of **alkalis, organic solvents**, and **sugar or salt solutions** (Figure 4.29) have been described as causing onycholysis.

In addition, there are infective causes.

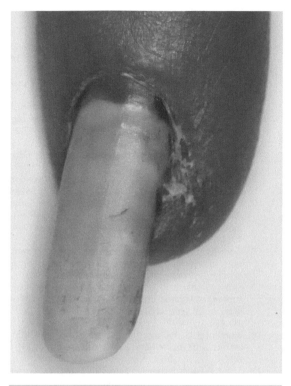

■ FIGURE 4.25

Onycholysis associated with a long natural nail (probably self-induced through lever action).

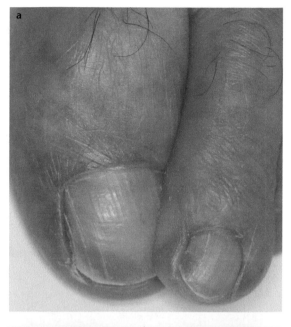

a

b

■ FIGURE 4.27

(a) Hidden lateral onycholysis of the big toenail due to overlapping. (b) Appearance of the onycholysis.

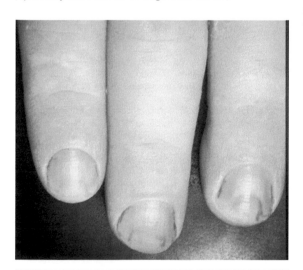

■ FIGURE 4.26

Onycholysis in a slaughterhouse worker. (Courtesy of T Menne, Denmark).

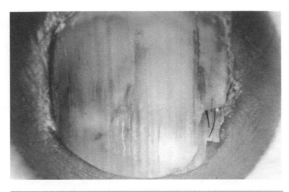

■ FIGURE 4.28

Onycholysis due to foreign bodies in a hairdresser.

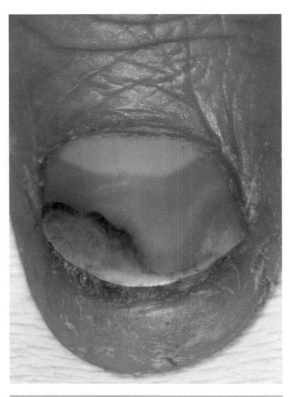

■ FIGURE 4.29

Onycholysis in an automotive worker (gas oil).

■■■ REFERENCES

1. Alkiewicz J, Majewski C. Clinical and histopathological features of onycholysis. Przegl Dermatol 1954; 41: 437–49. [in Polish]
2. Eastmond CJ, Wright V. The nail dystrophy of psoriatic arthritis. Ann Rheum Dis 1979; 38: 226–8.
3. Ray L. Onycholysis. Arch Dermatol Syph 1963; 88: 181.
4. Baran R, Badillet G. Primary onycholysis of the big toenails. A review of 113 cases. Br J Dermatol 1982; 106: 526–34.
5. Haneke E. Fungal infections of the nail. Sem Dermatol 1991; 10: 41–53.
6. Kechijian P. Onycholysis of the finger nails: evaluation and management. J Am Acad Dermatol 1985; 12: 552–60.
7. Hemmer W, Focke M, Wantke F, Götz M, Jarisch R. Allergic contact dermatitis to artificial fingernails prepared from UV light-cured acrylates. J Am Acad Dermatol 1996; 35: 377.
8. Guin JD, Baas K, Nelson-Adesokan P. Contact sensitization to cyanoacrylate adhesive as a cause of severe onychodystrophy. Int J Dermatol 1998; 37: 31–6.
9. Sinha A, Marsh R, Langtry J. Spontaneous regression of subungual keratoacanthoma with reossification of underlying distal lytic phalanx. Clin Exp Dermatol 2005; 30: 20–2.
10. Blumental G. Paronychia and pyogenic granuloma-like lesions with isotretinoin. J Am Acad Dermatol 1984; 10: 677–8.
11. Sass JO, Jakob-Solder B, Heitger A, Tzimas G, Sarcletti M. Paronychia with pyogenic granuloma in a child treated with indinavir: the retinoid-mediated side effect theory revisited. Dermatology 2000; 200: 40–2.
12. Gaylis N. Infliximab in the treatment of an HIV positive patient with Reiter's syndrome. J Rheumatol 2003; 30: 407–11.
13. Sato S. Iron deficiency: structural and microchemical changes in hair, nails, and skin. Semin Dermatol 1991; 10: 313–19.
14. Samman PD, White WF. The yellow nail syndrome. Br J Dermatol 1964; 76: 153.
15. Kandil E. Yellow nail syndrome. Int J Dermatol 1973; 12: 238–40.
16. Jacobsen FK, Abildtrup N, Laursen SO Brandrup F, Jensen NK. Acrokeratosis paraneoplastica (Bazex' syndrome). Arch Dermatol 1984; 120: 502–4.
17. Valdivielso M, Longo I, Suarez R, Huerta M, Lazaro P. Acrokeratosis paraneoplastica (Bazex syndrome). J Eur Acad Dermatol Venereol 2005; 19: 340–4.
18. Richert B, André J, Bourguignon R, de la Brassinne M. Hyperkeratotic nail discoid lupus erythematosus evolving towards systemic lupus erythematosus: therapeutic difficulties. J Eur Acad Dermatol Venereol 2004; 18: 728–30.

19. Faure M, Hermier C, Perrot H. Cutaneous reactions to propranolol. Ann Dermatol Venereol 1979; 106: 161.

20. Vanhooteghem O, Richert B, Vindevoghel A, et al. Subungual abscess: a new ungual side-effect related to docetaxel therapy. Br J Dermatol 2000; 143: 462–4.

21. Nicolopoulos J, Howard A. Docetaxel-induced nail dystrophy. Australas J Dermatol 2002; 43: 293–4.

22. Wasner G, Hilpert F, Schattschneider J, et al. Docetaxel-induced nail changes – a neurogenic mechanism: a case report. J Neurooncol 2002; 58: 167–74.

23. Ghetti E, Piraccini BM, Tosti A.. Onycholysis and subungual haemorrhages secondary to systemic chemotherapy (paclitaxel). J Eur Acad Dermatol Venereol 2003; 17: 459–60.

24. Maino KL, Norwood C, Stashower ME. Onycholysis with the appearance of a 'sunset' secondary to capecitabine. Cutis 2003; 72: 234–6.

25. Chiewchanvit S, Noppakun K, Kanchanarattanakorn K. Mucocutaneous complications of chemotherapy in 74 patients from Maharaj Nakorn Chiang Mai Hospital. J Med Assoc Thai 2004; 87: 508–14.

26. Gori S, Colozza M, Mosconi AM, et al. Phase II study of weekly paclitaxel and trastuzumab in anthracycline- and taxane-pretreated patients with *HER2*-overexpressing metastatic breast cancer. Br J Cancer 2004; 90: 36–40.

27. Tinio P, Bershad S, Levitt JO. Medical Pearl: Docetaxel-induced onycholysis. J Am Acad Dermatol 2005; 52: 350–1.

28. Speechly-Dick ME, Owen ER. Mitozantrone-induced onycholysis. Lancet 1988; i: 113.

29. Mitchell PL, Harvey VJ. Mitozantrone-induced onycholysis. Eur J Cancer 1992; 28: 243–4.

30. Creamer, JD, Mortimer PS, Powles TJ. Mitozantrone-induced onycholysis. A series of five cases. Clin Exp Dermatol 1995; 20: 459–61.

31. Makris A, Mortimer P, Powles TJ. Chemotherapy-induced onycholysis. Eur J Cancer 1996; 32A: 374–5.

32. Freiman A, Bouganin N, O'Brien EA. Mitozantrone-induced onycholysis associated with subungual abscesses, paronychia, and pyogenic granuloma. J Drugs Dermatol 2005; 4: 490–2.

33. Passier A, Smits-van Herwaarden A, van Puijenbroek E. Photo-onycholysis associated with the use of doxycycline. BMJ 2004; 329: 265.

34. Ortonne JP, Baran R. Photoonycholyse induite par la photochimiothérapie orale. Ann Dermatol Venereol 1978; 105: 887–8.

35. Bazex J, Baran R, Monbrun F, et al. Hereditary distal onycholysis – a case report. Clin Exp Dermatol 1990; 15: 146–8.

Chapter 5

Paronychia and pyogenic granuloma

Chronic paronychia, a red painful swelling of the periungual nail folds, is not observed frequently in psoriasis, except for patients treated with retinoids (especially etretinate). It is equivalent to psoriasis occurring at other skin sites. Ganor[1] found that 38% of his adult women patients and 10% of adult women control dermatology patients suffered from psoriasis. The diagnosis of psoriatic chronic paronychia is obvious when the disease presents in other localizations. It may be more difficult when paronychia is isolated (Figures 5.1–5.3). This condition is related to retention of the scales involving the undersurface of the proximal nail fold (PNF)

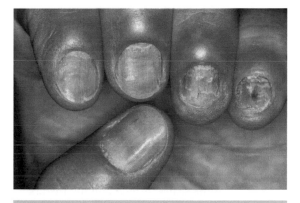

■ FIGURE 5.1

Recent psoriatic paronychia involving several fingers.

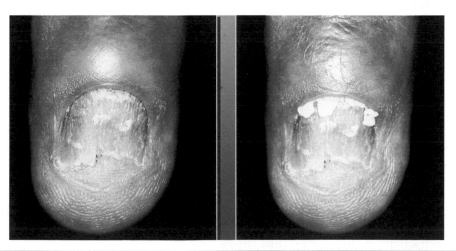

■ FIGURE 5.2

The same patient before and after squeezing the proximal nail fold.

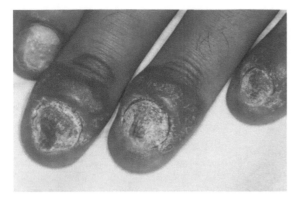

■ FIGURE 5.3

Advanced psoriatic chronic paronychia with totally dystrophic nails.

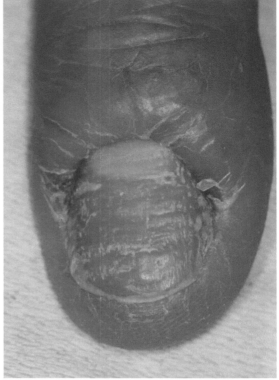

■ FIGURE 5.4

Allergic contact dermatitis in a housewife.

with a normal cuticle adherent to the dorsum of the nail plate. Gently squeezing the proximal nail fold leads to a discharge composed of clusters of keratinocytes with normal or pyknotic nuclei and anucleated cells. There are no inflammatory cells or fungal material, and a culture with Sabouraud's medium is negative. This suggests that the scales formed and retained beneath the PNF act as foreign bodies and incite the clinical response.

Depending on the major etiological factors involved,[2] the causes of chronic paronychia can be classified into a number of types (Table 5.1).

Contact allergy may be due to topical drug ingredients, rubber, etc. (Figure 5.4).

Food hypersensitivity may involve immediate protein contact dermatitis due to fruit, vegetables, spices, animal proteins, grains, enzymes (α-amylase in flour), or micro-organisms (Figure 5.5).

When the **hands are subjected to a moist envoironment**, paronychia may manifest as a red, semicircular indurated cushion around the base of the nail, which is detached from the distal portion of the PNF, with disappearance of the cuticle. This is followed by secondary retraction of the paronychial tissue. From time to time, the persistent low-grade inflammation may flare into subacute painful

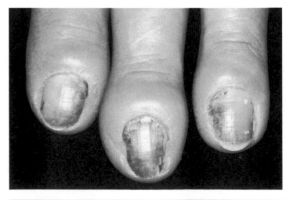

■ FIGURE 5.5

Food hypersensitivity in a housewife.

■ TABLE 5.1

Causes of paronychia

BACTERIAL

Classical

Erysipeloid

Leprosy

Milker's nodules

Mycobacterium marinum infection

Orf

Prosector's tuberculosis verrucosa cutis

Pseudomonas

Staphylococci

Streptococci

Syphilis

Tularemia

Unusual

Actinobacillus actinomycetemcomitans

Bartonella henselae

Corynebacterium spp. (in 10% of those affected by pitted keratolysis)

Eikenella corrodens

Klebsiella pneumoniae

Serratia marcescens

Torulopsis maris

FUNGAL

Aspergillus niger

Blastoschizomyces capitatus

Candida spp.

Curvularia lunata

Fusarium spp.

Microsporum gypseum

Scopulariopsis brevicaulis

Scytalidium spp.

Trichosporum beigelli

PARASITIC

Tungiasis

Leishmaniasis

VIRAL

Herpetic whitlow

DRUGS

5-Fluorouracil

Acitretin

Anti-epidermal growth factor receptor antibodies

Capecitabine

Cephalexin

Cetuximab

Gefitinib

Cyclophosphamide/vincristine

Cyclosporine

Docetaxel

Etretinate

Indinavir

Isotretinoin

Lamivudine

Methotrexate

Sirolimus

Sulfonamides

Zidovudine

DERMATOLOGICAL DISEASE

Artificial nails

Atopic dermatitis

Contact dermatitis

Darier's disease

Dyskeratosis congenita

Erythema multiforme

Finger-sucking (children)

Frostbite

Granulomas

Hidrotic ectodermal dysplasia

Ingrowing toenails

Leukemia cutis

Lichen planus

Pachyonychia congenita

Parakeratosis pustulosa

Causes of paronychia (*continued*)

DERMATOLOGICAL DISEASE (*continued*)

Pemphigoid, pemphigus

Pernio

Psoriasis

Radiodermatitis (chronic)

Reiter's disease

Rubinstein–Taybi syndrome

Stevens–Johnson syndrome

Repeated microtrauma

SYSTEMIC DISEASE

Acrodermatitis enteropathica

Acrokeratosis paraneoplastica

Chronic mucocutaneous candidiasis

Glucagonoma syndrome

Cushing syndrome

Diabetes mellitus

Digital ischemia

Epidemic encephalitis

Glioma

Graft-versus-host disease

Hypoparathyroidism

Immunosuppression

Job syndrome

Langerhans histiocytosis

Multiple mucosal neuroma syndrome

Neurofibroma

Neuropathies

Raynaud syndrome

Systemic lupus erythematosus

Sarcoidosis

Schwannoma

Systemic sclerosis

Systematized multiple fibrillar neuroma

Tricho-oculo-vertebral syndrome

Thromboangiitis obliterans

Wiscott–Aldrich syndrome

Yellow nail syndrome

Zinc deficiency

OCCUPATIONAL

Agricultural workers

Animal origin (bristles, sea urchins, oysters)

Automotive workers (sulfuric acid batteries)

Bakers and pastry cooks

Barbers and hairdressers (onycholysis)

Bartenders

Bean shellers

Bookbinders (paste)

Bricklayers (lime, cement, mortar)

Builders and carpenters (including glass fiber)

Button makers

Cement workers

Chemists and laboratory workers

Chicken factory workers

Cooks

Cosmetic workers

Dentists

Dinitrosalicylic acid

Dyers (aniline dyes, producing stains and necrosis)

Engravers (brittle nail)

Etchers, glass etchers (brittle nail)

Fishermen

Fishmongers

Florists and gardeners (onycholysis) (hyacinth, daffodil and narcissus bulbs, tulip fingers)

Glaziers (brittle nail)

Groundskeepers

Harpists

Housewives/husbands

Janitorial and domestic workers

Latex rubber

Manicurists (artificial nails)

Meat handlers

Mechanics

Milkers (onycholysis from bristles)

Oil-rig workers

Painters

■ TABLE 5.1
Causes of paronychia (*continued*)

OCCUPATIONAL (*continued*)	TUMORS (PRIMARY OR SECONDARY OF THE NAIL)
Photographic developers (brittle nail)	Bizarre parosteal osteochondroma of the tubular bones
Tanners (whitlow)	Bowen's disease
Textile workers (threads of fabric)	Enchondroma
Violinists (nail dystrophy)	Keratoacanthoma
Woodworkers (brittle nails, stains)	Melanoma
Woolworkers (wool thread)	Myxoid pseudocyst
	Osteoid osteoma

Reproduced with permission from Baran R, Dawber RPR, de Berker DAR, Haneke E, Tosti A, eds. Baran and Dawber's Diseases of the Nails and their Mangement, 3rd edn. Oxford: Blackwell Scientific, 2001.

exacerbation. This causes disturbances of the nail plate, with discolored, cross-ridged lateral edges, also reflecting *Candida* colonization (Figure 5.6). Consequently, true *Candida* paronychia is uncommon except in patients with chronic mucocutaneous candidiasis and HIV infection (Figure 5.7).

***Candida* hypersensitivity** exhibits a similar reaction to that suggested in some patients with recurrent vaginitis. In contrast to *Candida* infection, nondermatophyte molds such as *Fusarium* (Figure 5.8), *Aspergillus*, *Scytalidium* spp. (Figure 5.9), and even *Scopulariopsis brevicaulis* may produce **subacute paronychia**

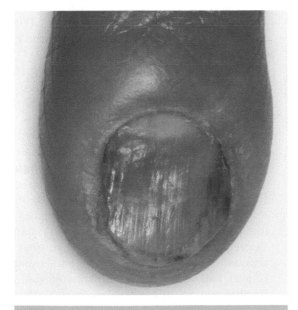

■ FIGURE 5.6

Candida colonization of chronic paronychia due to food hypersensitivity.

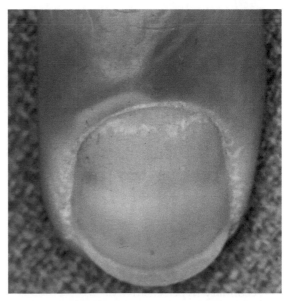

■ FIGURE 5.7

Subacute *Candida* paronychia in HIV infection. (Courtesy of BK Fisher, Ireland.)

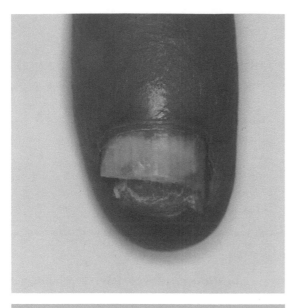

Subacute paronychia associated with *Fusarium* leukonychia.

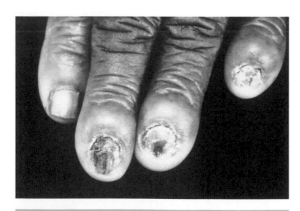

Chronic paronychia associated with *Scytalidium* infection.

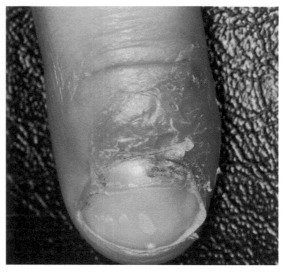

Staphylococcal infection.

accompanied by proximal white subungual onychomycosis.[3]

Irritant reactions may be associated with a secondary hypersensitivity.

Infections causing paronychia may be due to staphylococci (Figure 5.10), gram-negative cocci (Figures 5.11 and 5.12), tuberculosis (Figure 5.13), atypical *Mycobacterium marinum* infection (Figure 5.14), leprosy (Figure 5.15), primary syphilis (Figure 5.16), secondary syphilis (Figure 5.17), erysipeloid (Figure 5.18), parasites (*Tunga penetrans*) (Figure 5.19), herpes viruses (Figure 5.20), or warts on the ventral aspect of the PNF[4] (Figure 5.21).

Some drugs, such as retinoids, demonstrate a predilection for the paronychium and are responsible for paronychia (Figures 5.22 and 5.23) and/or pyogenic granuloma (Figures 5.24 and 5.25), involving toenails more often than fingernails.[5–7] In fact, these drugs produce a clinical and pathological condition indistinguishable from that of psoriatic chronic paronychia. Here also, the scales formed and retained at the undersurface of the PNF act as foreign bodies and induce a clinical inflammatory response. Consequently, like psoriatic paronychia, retinoid-induced paronychia has a similar pathogenesis, and the 'retinoid desquamative dermatitis' that appears in psoriatic patients is identical to the so-called 'psoriatic-like dermatitis' induced by etretinate in nonpsoriatic patients. Moreover, the high frequency of chronic parony-

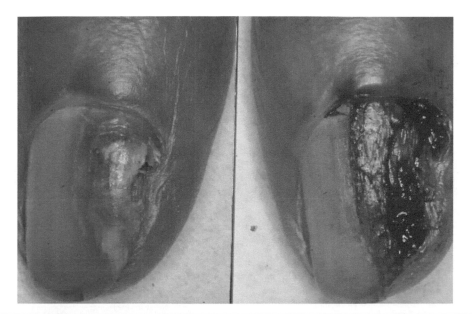

■ FIGURE 5.11

Pseudomonas infection.

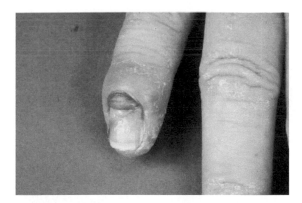

■ FIGURE 5.12

Coccal nail fold angiomatosis. (Courtesy of MG Davies, UK.)

chia in the group of psoriatics treated with etreti-nate compared with Darier's disease, for example, may be explained by an increase in the inflammatory response in psoriasis as an isomorphic phenomenon. In addition, psoriatic foci changing to paronychia have been repeatedly observed in psoriatics systemically treated with etretinate.

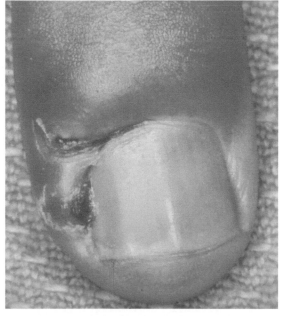

■ FIGURE 5.13

Prosector's paronychia tuberculosis infection. (Courtesy of D Goette, USA.)

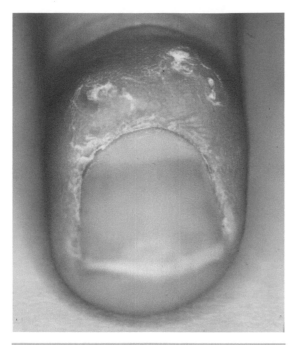

■ **FIGURE 5.14**

Paronychia in *Mycobacterium marinum* infection. (Courtesy of S Salasche, USA.)

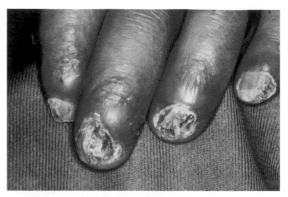

■ **FIGURE 5.15**

Paronychia in leprosy infection. (Courtesy of J Delacretaz, Switzerland.)

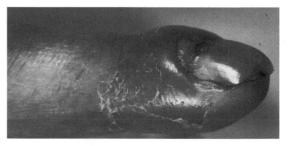

■ **FIGURE 5.16**

Primary syphilis involving the proximal nail fold. (Courtesy of J Garcia Silva, Spain.)

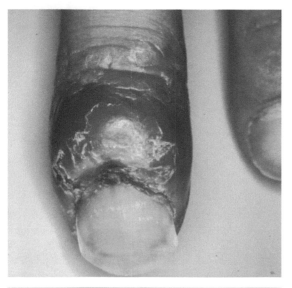

■ **FIGURE 5.17**

Secondary syphilis involving the proximal nail fold.

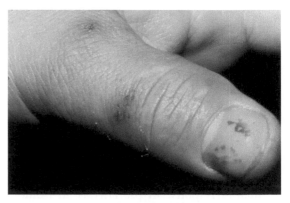

■ **FIGURE 5.18**

Erysipeloid infection involving the distal digit. (Courtesy of J Ortiz, Mexico.)

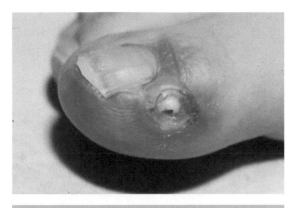

■ FIGURE 5.19

Tunga penetrans involving the nail fold. (Courtesy of C Zait, Brazil.)

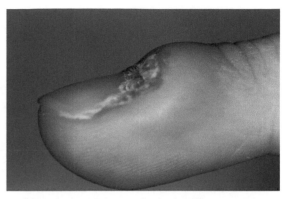

■ FIGURE 5.21

Warts involving the ventral aspect of the proximal nail fold. (Courtesy of A Eichmann, Switzerland.)

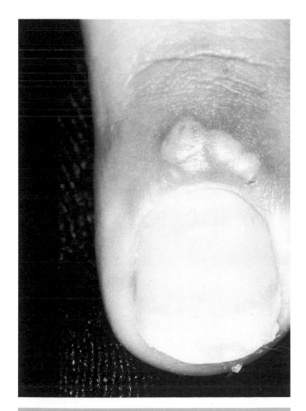

■ FIGURE 5.20

Paronychial vesiculous herpes virus infection.

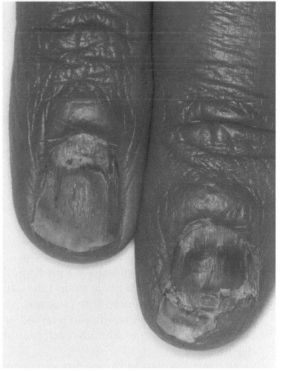

■ FIGURE 5.22

Subacute paronychia associated with nail dystrophy after etretinate therapy.

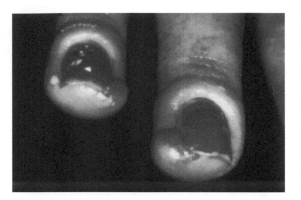

■ **FIGURE 5.23**

Paronychia associated with pyogenic granuloma due to etretinate. (Courtesy of L De Raeve, Belgium.)

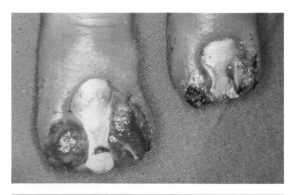

■ **FIGURE 5.24**

Pyogenic granuloma due to etretinate. (Courtesy of J Delescluse, Belgium.)

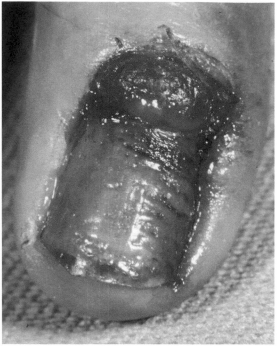

■ **FIGURE 5.25**

Pyogenic granuloma due to etretinate. (Courtesy of H Zaun, Germany.)

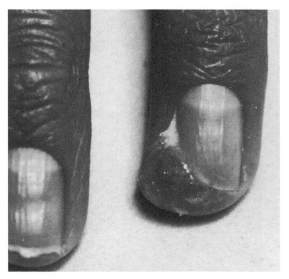

■ **FIGURE 5.26**

Pyogenic granuloma due to cyclosporine. (Courtesy of SH Wakelin, UK.)

In contrast to the usual appearance, where granulation tissue is rarely observed in fingernails, pyogenic granuloma may be seen in this area and usually indicates an iatrogenic origin.

Some patients probably have a predisposition to produce granulation tissue around the nails. A psoriatic patient presented with pyogenic granuloma after etretinate therapy and relapsed in the same areas when he was on cyclosporine[8-12] (Figure 5.26).

The pathogenesis of paronychia and pyogenic granuloma is unknown, but protease inhibitors may have a 'retinoid-like' effect due to homologies between the amino acid sequences of

CRABP1 and of the catalytic site of HIV-1 protease. Inhibition of endogenous proteases may explain the initial hypertrophy of the nail folds and the subsequent development of pyogenic granuloma-like lesions[13–18] (Figure 5.27). The mechanism of action of epidermal growth factor inhibitors may be similar.

The possibility that nail fold inflammation may represent an unusual reaction to fungi and bacteria has been demonstrated only in a case of severe paronychia due to zidovudine-induced neutropenia in a neonate.[19]

Acute paronychia has been reported with cephalexin[20] (Figure 5.28) and the **cytotoxic drugs** methotrexate,[21] and docetaxel[22] (Figure 5.29). Recently, **drugs targeting the epidermal growth factor receptor** (EGFR) have opened a new iatrogenic era associated with paronychial inflammation. Cetuximab (C225)[23,24] (an anti-EGFR antibody) and gefitinib[25,26] (an EGFR tyrosine kinase inhibitor) are both now being used as chemotherapic agents. The nail changes appear within 3 months. Sirolimus used in renal transplants acts as an epidermal growth factor responsible for pyogenic granuloma in 10% of the patients treated with this drug.[27]

Dermatological conditions associated with paronychia include lichen planus (Figure 5.30), Darier's disease, pachyonychia congenita, pemphigus vulgaris (Figure 5.31), and self-induced paronychia (Figure 5.32).

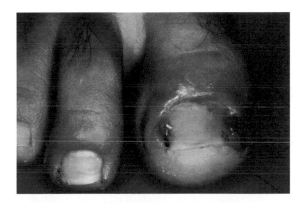

■ FIGURE 5.27

Paronychia and pyogenic granuloma due to protease inhibitors. (Courtesy of JP Morini, France.)

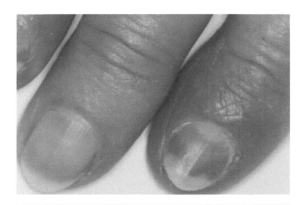

■ FIGURE 5.28

Acute paronychia after cephalexin.

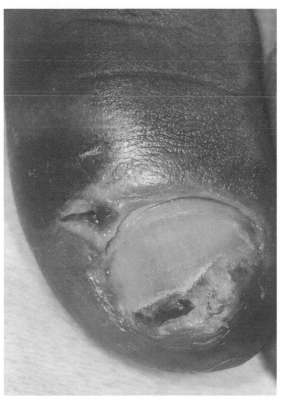

■ FIGURE 5.29

Subacute paronychia associated with onycholysis after docetaxel.

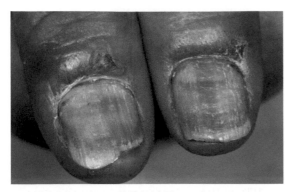

■ FIGURE 5.30

Chronic paronychia in lichen planus.

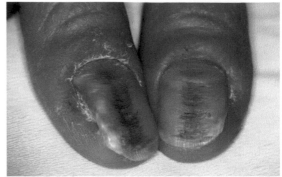

■ FIGURE 5.32

Self-induced paronychia (habit tic of pushing back the cuticle).

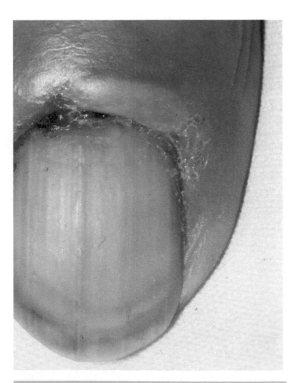

■ FIGURE 5.31

Paronychia in pemphigus vulgaris.

Paronychia not responding to medical therapy is probably *occupational*, and due to foreign bodies such as hair, bristle, or wood splinters (milkers, veterinarians, chefs, food handlers, and hairdressers)[28] (Figure 5.33).

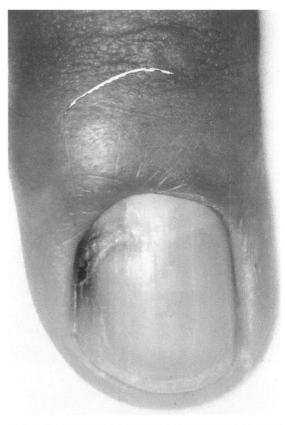

■ FIGURE 5.33

Chronic paronychia in a hairdresser (hair acts as foreign bodies).

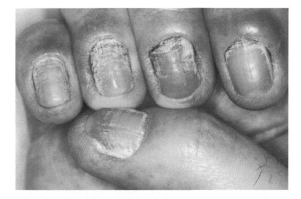

■ FIGURE 5.34

Yellow nail syndrome associated with paronychia.

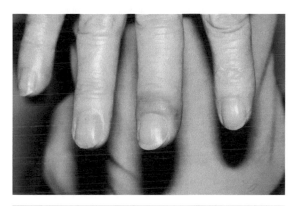

■ FIGURE 5.35

Sweet syndrome associated with subacute paronychia. (Courtesy of JP Callen, USA.)

Systemic diseases associated with paronychia include yellow nail syndrome (Figure 5.34), histiocytosis, Sweet syndrome (Figure 5.35), zinc deficiency (Figure 5.36), and gout.

Tumors of the nail apparatus and adjacent tissues (primary or secondary) may also cause paronychia.

■■■ REFERENCES

1. Ganor S. Diseases sometimes associated with psoriasis. I, Candidosis. Dermatologica 1977; 154: 268.
2. Tosti A, Piraccini PM, Ghetti E et al. Topical steroids versus systemic antifungals in the treatment of chronic paronychia. J Am Acad Dermatol 2002; 47: 73–6

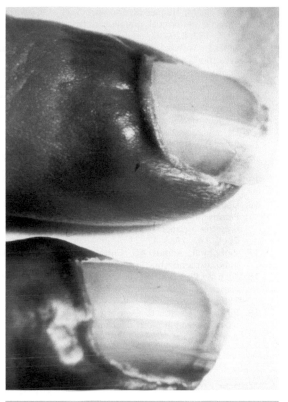

■ FIGURE 5.36

Subacute paronychia associated with zinc deficiency.

3. Baran R, Tosti A, Piraccini BM. Uncommon clinical patterns of *Fusarium* nail infection: report of three cases. Br J Dermatol 1997; 136: 424–7.
4. Lauchli S, Eichmann A, Baran R. Swelling of the proximal nail fold caused by underlying warts. Dermatology 2001; 202: 328–9.
5. Baran R. Etretinate and the nails (study of 130 cases): possible mechanisms of some side effects. Clin Exp Dermatol 1986; 11: 148–52.
6. De Raeve L, Willemsen M, De Coninck A et al. Paronychie et formation de tissu granuleux au cours d'un traitement par isotretinoine. Dermatologica 1986; 172: 278–80.
7. Blumental G. Paronychia and pyogenic granuloma-like lesions with isotretinoin. J Am Acad Dermatol 1984; 4: 677–8
8. Wakelin SH, Emmerson RW. Excess granulation tissue development during treatment with cyclosporin. Br J Dermatol 1994; 131: 147–8.
9. Olujohungbe A, Cox J, Hammon MD et al. Ingrowing toenails and cyclosporin. Lancet 1993; 342: 1111.
10. Dandurand M, El Mejjaoui S, Guillot B. Bourgeons charnus, ongles incarnés et ciclosporine. Ann Dermatol Venereol 1999; 26 (2S): 158–9.

11. Higgins EM, Hugues JR, Snowden S, et al. Cyclosporin-induced periungual granulation tissue. Br J Dermatol 1995; 132: 829–30.

12. Tanaka, Yoshikawa N, Kitano Y, et al. Long term cyclosporin treatment in children with steroid-dependent nephrotic syndrome. Paediatr Nephrol 1993; 7: 249–52.

13. Sass JO, Jakob-Sölder B, Heitger A et al. Paronychia with pyogenic granuloma in a child treated with Indinavir : the retinoid-mediated side effect theory revisited. Dermatology 2000; 200: 40–2.

14. Bouscarat F, Bouchard C, Bouhour D. Paronychia and pyogenic granuloma of the great toes in patients treated with indinavir. N Engl J Med 1998; 338: 1776–7.

15. Alam M, Scher RK. Indinavir-related recurrent paronychia and ingrown toenails. Cutis 1999; 64: 277–8.

16. Dauden E, Pascual-Lopez M, Martinez-Garcia C, et al. Paronychia and excess granulation tissue of the toes and finger in a patient treated with indinavir. Br J Dermatol 2000; 142: 1063–4.

17. Zerboni R, Angius AG, Cusini M, et al. Lamivudine-induced paronychia. Lancet 1998; 351: 1256.

18. Tosti A, Piraccini BM, D'Antuono A, et al. Paronychia associated with antiretroviral therapy. Br J Dermatol 1999; 140: 1165–8.

19. Russo F, Collantes C, Guerrero J. Severe paronychia due to zidovudine-induced neutropenia in a neonate. J Am Acad Dermatol 1999; 40: 322–4.

20. Baran R, Perrin C. Fixed drug eruption presenting as an acute paronychia. Br J Dermatol 1991; 125: 592–5.

21. Wantzin GL, Thomsen K. Acute paronychia after high-dose methotrexate therapy. Arch Dermatol 1983; 119: 623–4.

22. Correia O, Azevedo C, Pinto-Ferreira E, et al. Nail changes secondary to docetaxel (Taxotere). Dermatology 1999; 198: 288–90

23. Boucher KW, Davidson K, Mirakhur B et al. Paronychia induced by cetuximab, an antiepidermal growth factor receptor antibody. J Am Acad Dermatol 2002; 45: 632–3

24. Busam KJ, Capodieci P, Motzer R et al. Cutaneous side-effects in cancer patients treated with the antiepidermal growth factor receptor antibody C225. Br J Dermatol 2001; 144: 1169–76.

25. Nakano J, Nakamura M. Paronychia induced by gefitinib, an epidermal growth factor receptor tyrosine kinase inhibitor. J Dermatol 2003; 30: 261–2.

26. Dainichi T, Tanaka M, Tsuruta N et al. Development of multiple paronychia and periungual granulation in patients treated with gefitinib, an inhibitor of epidermal growth factor receptor. Dermatology 2003; 207: 324–5.

27. Mahé E, Morelon E, Lechaton S, et al. Onychopathie associée au sirolimus. Poster 84. Ann Dermatol Venereol 2005; 132 (9S): 121.

28. Baran R, Bureau H. Surgical treatment of recalcitrant chronic paronychia of fingers. J Dermatol Surg Oncol 1981; 7:106–7.

Chapter 6

Nail discoloration

Nail discoloration indicates an abnormality in the color of the fabric and/or surface of the nail and/or subungual tissue. Discoloration may result from abnormalities of the nail plate itself, abnormalities at the nail plate–nail bed attachment (onycholysis or subungual hyperkeratosis), and abnormalities of the nail bed.

In patients whose nails are in contact occupationally with coloring chemicals or after topical application of therapeutic agents, neither fingertip pressure producing blanching nor a pen-torch placed against the pulp will alter the discoloration, which most often follows the shape of the proximal nail fold when it grows out (Figure 6.1).

When melanocytic pigmentation or non-melanocytic hyperchromia involve all of the digits and follow the shape of the lunula (Figure 6.2), it may result from the systemic absorption of a drug or a chemical through the lung or the skin. This discoloration of the nail has two different origins:

1. Disappearance of the dyschromia on the nail bed blanching test means that the coloration originates from the blood vessels.
2. If the dyschromia is not altered on the nail bed blanching test, but is obliterated by a pen-torch pressed against the pulp, then the pigment or the nonmelanocytic hyperchromia is deposited in the nail bed tissue.

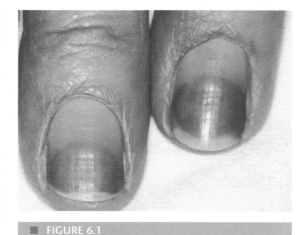

■ FIGURE 6.1

Exogenous discoloration follows the shape of the proximal nail fold.

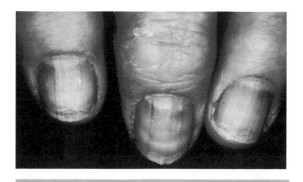

■ FIGURE 6.2

Endogenous discoloration after systemic drug absorption follows the shape of the lunula.

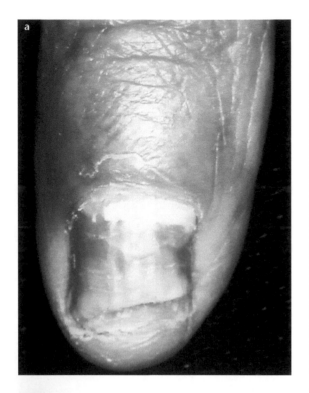

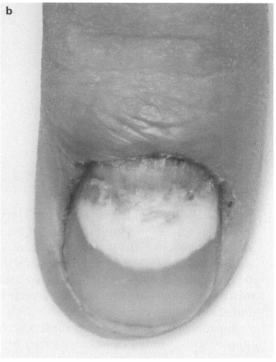

(a) Psoriatic transverse leukonychia. (b) Psoriatic white patch following the shape of the lunula. (c) Psoriatic total leukonychia.

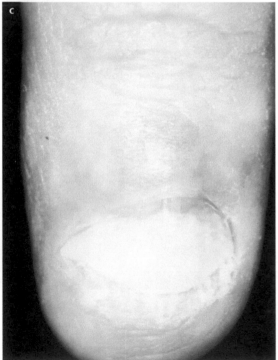

■■■ LEUKONYCHIA

In psoriasis, the nail may be affected by true leukonychia, due to involvement of the distal matrix as a transverse band (Figure 6.3) or large patches[1] and apparent leukonychia (Figure 6.4), due to onycholysis and/or to parakeratotic deposits in the nail bed leading to subungual hyperkeratosis. The parakeratotic cells filling the pits of the dorsum of the nail usually disappear quickly when they come from beneath the proximal nail fold. However, these cells may adhere to each other, producing a superficial white friable nail plate called pseudoleukonychia (Figure 6.5).

In addition to the distal involvement, sometimes a pathological process may also affect the

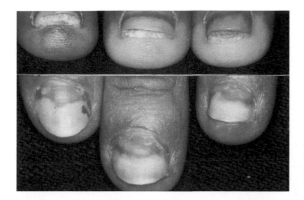

■ FIGURE 6.4

Psoriatic apparent leukonychia due to subungual hyperkeratosis.

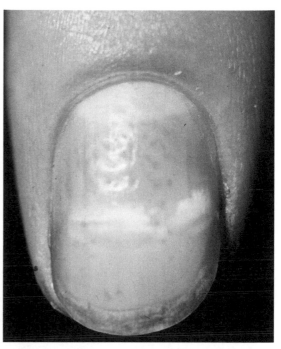

■ FIGURE 6.6

Associated psoriatic pitting and transverse leukonychia.

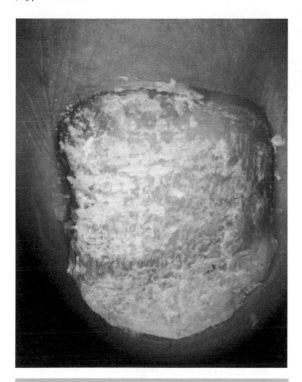

■ FIGURE 6.5

Psoriatic pseudoleukonychia. (Courtesy of B Schubert, France.)

proximal portion of the matrix, producing associated pitting and usually signaling a diagnosis of psoriasis in cases restricted to the nail (Figure 6.6).

Onychomycosis presents with similar changes, namely transverse leukonychia in the proximal white subungual type (Figure 6.7), and patches or even total leukonychia (Figure 6.8) in distal subungual onychomycosis and in superficial white onychomycosis (Figure 6.9).

However, alopecia areata may present with almost identical features, namely transverse leukonychia, sometimes associated with pitting or trachyonychia (see Chapter 1).

Generally speaking, white nails are the most common chromatic nail abnormality, and these can be divided into three main types: **true leukonychia**, where nail plate involvement originates in the matrix, **apparent leukonychia**, with involvement of the nonmatrix subungual tissue, and **pseudoleukonychia**.

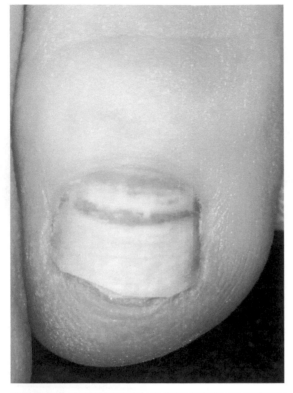

■ FIGURE 6.7

Proximal white subungual onychomycosis due to *Fusarium*.

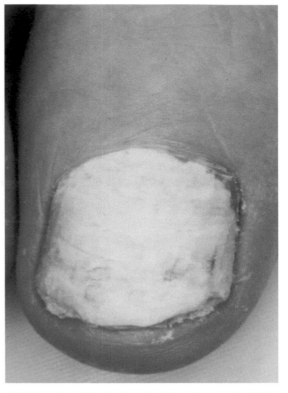

■ FIGURE 6.8

Distal subungual onychomycosis due to *Trichophyton rubrum*.

■■■ TRUE LEUKONYCHIA

Congenital forms of leukonychia are mainly transmitted as autosomal dominant traits (Table 6.1). They are usually total or subtotal, and are rarely punctate or striate. These congenital forms can be associated with other malformations of the nail, skin, or other tissue (e.g. deafness). All 20 digits are usually involved, but sometimes only the fingers are affected.

Acquired forms may be exogenous or endogenous (Table 6.2).

■ TOTAL LEUKONYCHIA

In this rare condition, the nail may be milky, chalky, bluish, ivory, or porcelain white in color

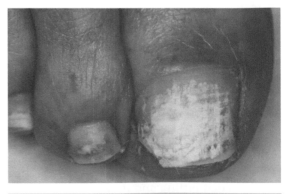

■ FIGURE 6.9

Superficial white onychomycosis due to *Aspergillus*.

■ TABLE 6.1

Conditions with congenital and/or hereditary discoloration of nails listed according to color changes

Disease	Appearance of nail	Inheritance[a]	Comments and references
Keratitis, ichthyosis, and deafness	White, thick	AR 242150	KID syndrome [46]
Keratoderma palmoplantare with atrophic fibrosis of extremities	White	AD 181600	[47]
Leopard syndrome	White with koilonychia	AD *151100	Lentigines, electrocardiographic changes, ocular hypertelorism, pulmonary stenosis, abnormalities of genitalia, retarded growth, deafness[48]
Leukonychia totalis	Milky or porcelain	AD *151600	[49]
Leukonychia totalis plus epiphyseal dysplasia (Lowry–Wood) syndrome	Milky	AR *226960	Also nystagmus, hypoplasia of corpus callosum, microcephaly[50]
Leukonychia subtotalis	Milky or porcelain	AD *151600	Pink area (2–4 mm), distal to white area
Striate leukonychia	Milky or porcelain	AD	Longitudinal or transverse band[51]
Striate leukonychia plus eruptive milia	Milky or porcelain		
Leukonychia plus koilonychia	Milky or porcelain	AD	[52]
Leukonychia plus koilonychia plus deafness plus knuckle pads plus keratoderma palmoplantare	Milky or porcelain	AD *149200	[53]

Conditions with congenital and/or hereditary discoloration of nails listed according to colour changes (*continued*)

Disease	Appearance of nail	Inheritance[a]	Comments and references
Leukonychia plus multiple sebaceous cysts plus renal calculi (FLOTCH syndrome)	Milky or porcelain	AD	54,55
Leukonychia plus onychorrhexis plus hypoparathyroidism plus dental changes plus cataract	Milky or porcelain	AR	56
Leukonychia plus duodenal ulcer plus gallstones	Milky or porcelain	?	57
Leukonychia plus pili torti	White		58
Acrokeratosis verruciformis (Hopf's disease)	White in early years. Brown with ridging and subungual hyperkeratosis in later life	AD *101900	Verrucous or lichenoid papules on the dorsa of hands and fingers. Palms and soles may be involved as translucent punctae[59]
Hemochromatosis	White, gray, or brownish	AD *235200	Periungual area brown. Koilonychia in 50%

Reproduced with permission from Baran R, Dawber RPR, de Berker DAR, Haneke E, Tosti A, eds. Baran and Dawber's Diseases of the Nails and their Management, 3rd edn. Oxford: Blackwell Science, 2001.

[a]MIM (Mendelian Inheritance in Man) number; AR, autosomal recessive; AD, autosomal dominant.

(Figure 6.10). The opacity of the whiteness varies. When it is faintly opaque, it may be possible to see transverse streaks of leukonychia in a nail with total leukonychia. Involvement of the longitudinal half of the nail plate has been described in a patient presenting with total leukonychia in some other digits.

Accelerated nail growth is associated with total leukonychia.

Kates et al[2] presented the pedigree of a family with 28 affected members.

■ SUBTOTAL LEUKONYCHIA

In this form, there is a pink arc about 2–4 mm wide distal to the white area.[3] This can be explained by the fact that the nucleated cells in the distal area mature, lose their keratohyalin granules, and then produce healthy keratin several weeks after they have been formed. The possibility that there are parakeratotic cells along the whole length of the nail has been discussed. These decrease in number as they approach the

■ **TABLE 6.2**

Etiology of leuconychia

CONGENITAL AND/OR HEREDITARY

Isolated or associated with other conditions

ACQUIRED

Pseudoleukonychia

Frictional cause (toenails)

2-Ethyl-cryanoacrylate glue

Keratin granulation (nail varnish, base-coat)

Onychomycosis

Psoriasis

Apparent leukonychia

Anemia

Cancer chemotherapeutic agents

Cirrhosis

Fly-tyer's finger

Half-and-half nail, distal crescent pigmentation (renal disease, androgen, 5-fluorouracil)

Leprosy

Muehrcke's lines with hypoalbuminemia or normal albuminemia (trauma, aging)

Ulcerative colitis

Peptic ulcer disease and cholelithiasis

Psoriasis

True leukonychia

Alkaline metabolic disease

Acute rejection of renal allograft

Altitude leukonychia

Alopecia areata

Breast cancer

Cachectic state

Carcinoid tumors of the bronchus

Cardiac insufficiency

Crow–Fukase syndrome (POEMS)

Cytotoxic and other drugs (emetine, pilocarpine sulfonamides, cortisone, quinacrine, trazodone)

Dyshidrosis

Endemic typhus

Erythema multiforme

Exfoliative dermatitis

Fasting periods in orthodox Jews

Fracture

Gout

Hodgkin's disease

Hyperalbuminemia

Hypocalcemia

Immunohemolytic anemia

Infectious diseases and infectious fevers

Intra-abdominal malignancies

Kawasaki syndrome

Kidney transplant

Leuko-onycholysis paradentotica

Leprosy

Lichen planopilaris

Malaria

Malnutrition and myoedema

Menstrual cycle

Myocardial infarction

Nitric acid, nitrite solution

Occupational

Parasitic infestations

Pellagra

Peripheral neuropathy

Pneumonia

Poisoning (antimony, arsenic, carbon monoxide, fluoride, lead, thallium)

Protein deficiency

Psoriasis

Psychotic episodes (acute)

Renal failure (acute or chronic)

Rickettsia

Salt plant workers

Shock

Sickle cell anemia

Surgery

■ TABLE 6.2	
Etiology of leuconychia (*continued*)	
Sympathetic leukonychia	Vascular impairment
Systemic lupus erythematosus	Zinc deficiency
Trauma (repeated)	Zoster
Trichinosis	

Reproduced with permission from Baran R, Dawber RPR, de Berker DAR, Haneke E, Tosti A, eds. Baran and Dawber's Diseases of the Nails and their Management, 3rd edn. Oxford: Blackwell Science, 2001.

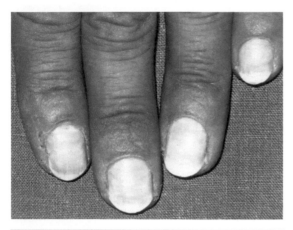

■ FIGURE 6.10

Congenital total leukonychia.

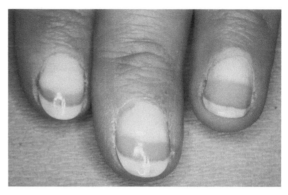

■ FIGURE 6.11

Congenital subtotal leukonychia.

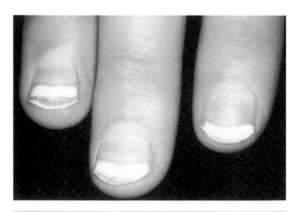

■ FIGURE 6.12

Congenital transverse leukonychia.

distal end, thus producing the normal pink color up to the point of separation from the nail bed. There might, however, be enough of these cells left for the nail to acquire a whitish tint when it has lost contact with the nail bed.

In subtotal (Figure 6.11) or even total leukonychia, proximal subungual onychomycosis and trauma to the proximal nail fold have to be ruled out.

■ TRANSVERSE LEUKONYCHIA

Besides congenital forms (Figure 6.12), one or several nails may exhibit a band, usually transverse, 1–2 mm wide, and single or occurring at the same level in each nail. This results, for example, from retinoids, acute arsenic toxicity (Mees' lines) (Figure 6.13), cytotoxic drugs (Figure 6.14), trauma, repeated microtrauma resulting from lack of trimming and impingment on the distal part of a shoe[4] (Figure 6.15), or acute rejection of

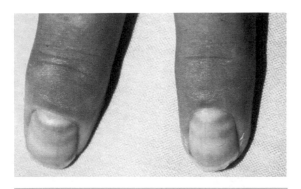

■ FIGURE 6.13

Mees' lines (arsenic toxicity).

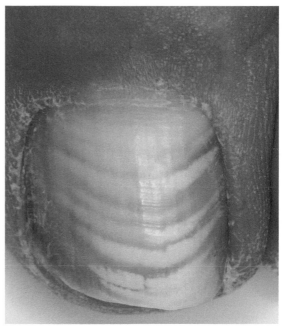

■ FIGURE 6.15

Multiple transverse leukonychia resulting from repeated microtrauma on the free margin of the nail.

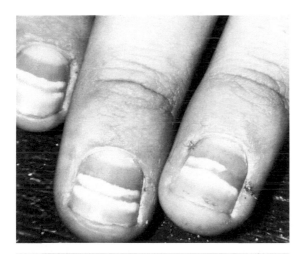

■ FIGURE 6.14

Transverse leukonychia due to cytotoxic drug.

a renal allograft.[5] Proximal white subungual onychomycosis has to be ruled out (Figure 6.7).

■ PUNCTATE LEUKONYCHIA

In this type, white spots 1–3 mm in diameter (Figure 6.16) occur singly or in groups;[6] only rarely do they occur on toenails. Their appearance is usually due to repeated minor trauma to the matrix. The evolution of the spots is variable; appearing generally on contact with the cuticle, they grow distally with the nail, but about half

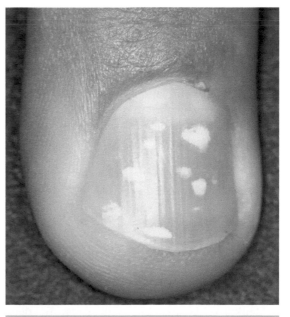

■ FIGURE 6.16

Punctate leukonychia.

of them disappear in the course of their migration toward the free edge. This proves that parakeratotic cells are capable of maturing and losing their keratohyalin granules to produce keratin, even though they have been without vascularization for many months. Some white spots enlarge, while others appear at a distance from the lunula, suggesting that the nail bed is participating by incorporating groups of nucleated cells into the nail. A similar process could explain the exclusively distal leukonychia that is occasionally seen. A local or general fault in normal keratinization is not the only cause of punctate leukonychia. Infiltration of air, which is known to occur in cutaneous parakeratoses, may also play a part.

Leukonychia punctata may be seen in psoriasis and in alopecia areata, where the shallow pits are sometimes lined with residual adherent parakeratotic cells.

■ LONGITUDINAL LEUKONYCHIA (Figure 6.17)

Longitudinal leukonychia is characterized by a permanent grayish-white longitudinal streak, 1 mm wide, below the nail plate. Histologically, there is a mound of horny cells causing the white discoloration due to a lack of transparency resulting in an alteration in light diffraction. Early stages of longitudinal splits and ridges of the nail may appear as white streaks. They may represent Darier's disease[7] or Hailey–Hailey disease. Epidermal hamartoma presenting as longitudinal pachyleukonychia restricted to fingernails has been reported.[8]

■■■ APPARENT LEUKONYCHIA

Any type of onycholysis may produce apparent leukonychia, as well as parakeratotic deposits in the nail bed. This may be observed in onychomycosis.

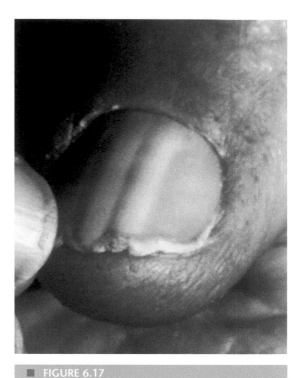

■ **FIGURE 6.17**

Longitudinal leukonychia.

■ TERRY'S NAIL

This presents as a white opacity of the nails in patients with cirrhosis. In the majority of cases, the nails are opaque and white, obscuring the lunula. This discoloration, which stops suddenly 1–2 mm from the distal edge of the nail, leaves a pink to brown area 0.5–3.0 mm wide that is not obscured by venous congestion and corresponds to the onychocorneal band.[9] It lies parallel to the distal part of the nail bed and may be irregular (Figure 6.18). The condition involves all nails uniformly. A revised definition and new correlations of Terry's nails have been advocated by Holzberg and Walker.[10] They found that a distal brown band was four times more frequent than the normal pink band as described by Terry. The proximal nail beds of one-quarter of the patients were light pink, rather than white, with a ground-glass opacity. The nail abnormality is associated with cirrhosis, and associations have

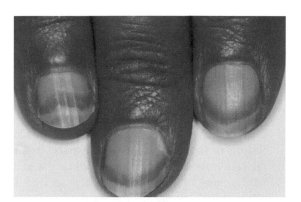

■ FIGURE 6.18

Terry's nails.

been demonstrated with chronic congestive heart failure, adult-onset diabetes mellitus, and age.

■ UREMIC HALF-AND-HALF NAIL

This nail consists of two segments separated more or less transversely by a well-defined line;[11] the proximal area is dull white, resembling ground glass and obscuring the lunula; the distal area is pink, reddish, or brown, and occupies 20–60% of the total length of the nail (average 33%) (Figure 6.19). In typical cases, diagnosis

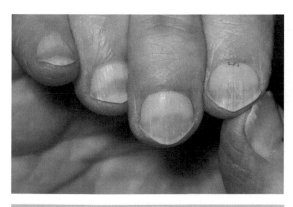

■ FIGURE 6.19

Uremic half-and-half nail.

presents no difficulty, but in Terry's nail, the pink, distal area may occupy up to 50% of the length of the nail, in which case the two types of nail may be confused. Half-and-half nail can display a normal proximal half portion, and the color of the distal part can be due either to an increase in the number of capillaries and thickening of their walls or to melanin granules in the nail bed. Sometimes, the distinctly abnormal onychodermal band extends approximately 20–25% from the distal portion of the fingernail as a distal crescent of pigmentation with pigment throughout the brown arc of the nail plate.[12] Half-and-half nails have occurred after chemotherapy.[13]

■ MUEHRCKE'S PAIRED, NARROW WHITE BANDS[14]

These bands, which are parallel to the lunula, are separated from one another, and from the lunula, by strips of pink nail (Figure 6.20). They

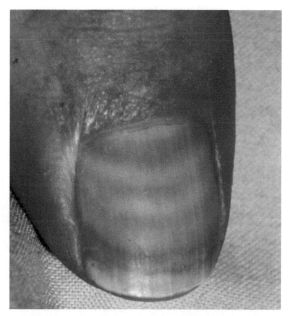

■ FIGURE 6.20

Muehrcke's paired, narrow white bands. (Courtesy of K Thomson, Denmark.)

disappear when the serum albumin level returns to normal and reappear if it falls again. However, white fingernails preceded by multiple transverse white bands have been reported with normal serum albumin levels. Cytotoxic drugs may produce Muehrcke's bands. Unilateral Muehrcke's bands may even develop after trauma.[15]

Nail changes similar to those reported above have been termed 'Neapolitan nail' in the elderly:[16] they are probably simply an age-related phenomenon.

■ ANEMIA

Anemia produces a pallor with apparent leukonychia.

■ PSEUDOLEUKONYCHIA

Besides the parakeratotic cells filling the pits in psoriasis and even alopecia areata and the subungual types of onychomycosis, the differential diagnosis of pseudoleukonychia includes superficial white onychomycosis (Figure 6.9), cosmetic keratin granulation[17] (Figure 6.21) and frictional worn-out nail involving especially the big toe (Figure 6.22). Surface pseudoleukonychia is responsible for superficial friability. Leukonychia from 2-ethylcyanoacrylate glue application

is associated with microfractures in the intermediate portion of the nail plate.[18]

■■■ OIL SPOTS (SALMON SPOTS)

Oily patches originate from circumscribed lesions of the nail bed. They are associated with an exudative inflammation producing a yellowish hue due to glycoprotein of the serum.[1] They are especially typical of the psoriatic nail (Figure 6.23).

Less commonly, they occur in acrodermatitis continua suppurativa and in systemic lupus erythematosus.[1] Very large patches have been described in lectitis purulenta et granulomatosa (granulomatous purulent nail bed inflammation).[19,20]

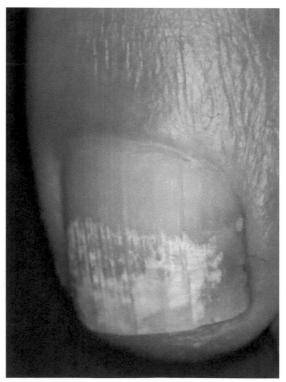

■ FIGURE 6.22

Frictional worn-out big toenail.

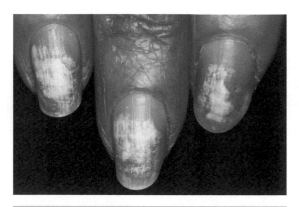

■ FIGURE 6.21

Cosmetic keratin granulation.

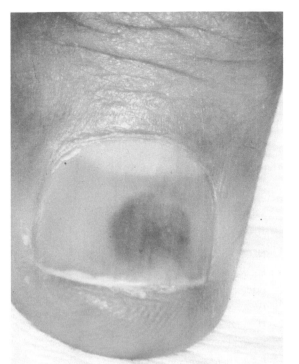

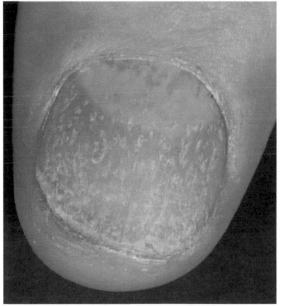

FIGURE 6.24

Spotted red lunula in psoriasis.

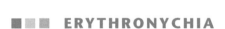

FIGURE 6.23

Oily spot. (Reproduced from Baran and Dawber. Diseases of the Nails, 3rd ed. Oxford: Blackwell Science, 2001, with kind permission of Blackwell Science.)

■■■ ERYTHRONYCHIA

■ RED LUNULA

The half-moon of the nails, which is usually of a ground-glass appearance, may become reddened or suffused. Dusky red, blanchable erythema of the lunula can be observed in psoriasis (Figure 6.24). Spotting and mottling of the lunula has been noted by Shelley.[21] The lunula develops small, discrete lacunae or plaques in which the white color is absent, giving a mottled or motheaten appearance. They are reversible.

Among the causes of red lunulae (Table 6.3), the most frequent dermatological conditions presenting with this characteristic are alopecia areata[22] (Figure 6.25) and lichen planus (Figure 6.26). Purpura in the lunula has also been

FIGURE 6.25

Red mottled lunula associated with trachonychia in alopecia areata. (Courtesy of M Pasch, The Netherlands.)

reported. Red lunulae occur mainly in congestive heart failure[23] (Figure 6.27), although they can also be observed in patients with many other cutaneous (Figure 6.28) and systemic (Figure 6.29) disorders or may be idiopathic.

■ TABLE 6.3

Disorders in patients with red lunulae

CARDIOVASCULAR

Angina pectoris

Atherosclerotic disease

Conduction abnormality

Congestive heart failure

Fever-induced heart disease

Hypertension

Myocardial infarction

DERMATOLOGICAL

Alopecia areata

Chronic urticaria

Dermatomyositis

Lichen sclerosus et atrophicus

Lupus erythematosus

Psoriasis vulgaris

20-nail dystrophy

Vitiligo

ENDOCRINE

Diabetes mellitus

Hyperthyroidism

Not specified

Thyroid disease

GASTROINTESTINAL

Esophageal strictures

Irritable bowel syndrome

Pyloric channel ulcer

HEPATIC

Cirrhosis

HEMATOLOGICAL

Anemia of chronic disease

Idiopathic transient leukopenia

INFECTIOUS

Lymphogranuloma venereum

Pneumonia

Tuberculosis

MISCELLANEOUS

Alcohol abuse

Carbon monoxide poisoning

Chronic idiopathic lymphedema

Corticosteroid therapy and other drugs

Hay fever pollen desensitization

Malnutrition

Senile macular degeneration

Tobacco abuse

Trauma and repeated microtrauma (habit tic)

NEOPLASTIC

Enchondroma

Hodgkin's disease

Lymphoid follicular reticulosis

Lymphosarcoma

Myeloid leukemia

Polycythemia vera

Reticulosarcoma

Submatrix pseudomyxoid cyst

NEUROLOGICAL

Cerebrovascular accident

PULMONARY

Chronic bronchitis

Chronic obstructive pulmonary disease

Emphysema

RENAL

Proteinuria

RHEUMATOLOGICAL

Baker's cyst (degenerative)

Osteoarthritis

Polymyalgia rheumatica

Rheumatoid arthritis

Reproduced with permission from Baran R, Dawber RPR, de Berker DAR, Haneke E, Tosti A, eds. Baran and Dawber's Diseases of the Nails and their Management, 3rd edn. Oxford: Blackwell Science, 2001.

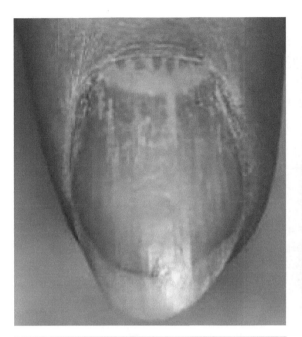

■ **FIGURE 6.26**

Red mottled lunula in alopecia areata.

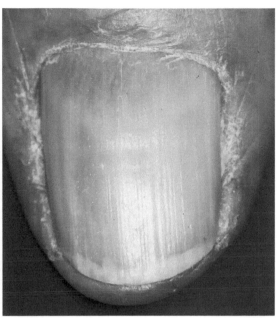

■ **FIGURE 6.27**

Red lunula in congestive heart failure.

■ LONGITUDINAL ERYTHRONYCHIA

Longitudinal erythronychia is rarely observed in the psoriatic nail bed (Figure 6.30), but a red longitudinal streak may be seen through the nail plate in a range of disorders and patterns (Table 6.4).

The red band, either single (Figure 6.31) or double (Figure 6.32), may be replaced by a linear hemorrhage or an interrupted line, composed of splinter hemorrhages. Associated with distal nail bed onychopapilloma,[24] this type of longitudinal erythronychia may be a marker for Bowen's disease,[25] in contrast to the idiopathic polydactylous type[26] (Figure 6.33).

■ RED/PURPLE NAIL BED

Besides the redness surrounding proximally a psoriatic onycholytic area, a red nail bed usually results from drugs (clofazimine, heparin, war-

farin, capecitabine, or PUVA), from polycythemia, or from vascular tumors such as hemangiomas[27] (Figure 6.34), glomus tumors (Figure 6.35), subungual arteriovenous tumors,[28] angiolymphoid hyperplasia with eosinophilia[29] (Figure 6.36), telangiectasia (Coat syndrome), or Rendu–Osler–Weber syndrome.[30] Transient subungual erythema has been reported in a patient with idiopathic Sweet syndrome, in contrast to the course of the half-and-half nail, where erythema is permanent.[31]

■■■ NONMELANOCYTIC HYPERCHROMIA

■ SPLINTER HEMORRHAGES

Splinter hemorrhages (Figure 6.37) are seen in the fingernails of 42% of psoriatics with nail disease and in the toenails of 6%.[32] The sign reflects the orientation of the capillary plexuses in the

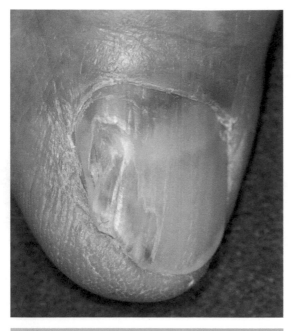

■ FIGURE 6.28

Submatricial myxoid pseudocyst showing red lunula.

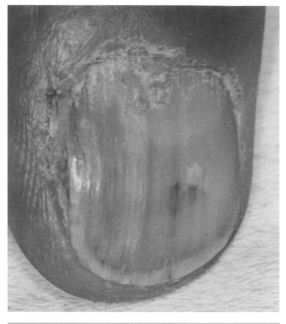

■ FIGURE 6.30

Longitudinal erythronychia. Multiple lines in psoriatic nail bed.

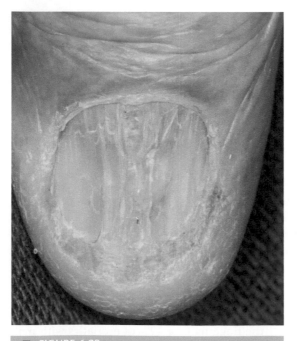

■ FIGURE 6.29

Red lunula in amyloidosis.

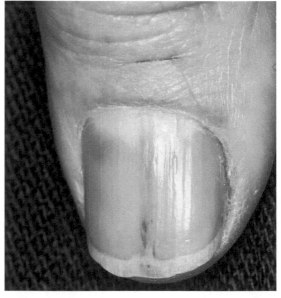

■ FIGURE 6.31

Idiopathic longitudinal erythronychia. (Reproduced from Baran and Perrin. Br J Dermatol 2000; 143: 132–5 with kind permission.)

■ **TABLE 6.4**

Causes of longitudinal erythronychia

ACANTHOLYTIC DYSKERATOSIS

Acantholytic epidermolysis bullosa[60]

Acantholytic naevus[61]

Darier's disease[7]

Warty dyskeratoma[62,63]

DERMATOLOGICAL CONDITION

Acrokeratosis verruciformis[62]

Bilobed thumbnail with erythronychia[64]

Factitious onychodystrophy[65]

Lichen planus

Psoriasis

SYSTEMIC DISEASE

Amyloidosis

Hemiplegia[66]

Pseudo-bulbar syndrome[67]

LOCAL BENIGN TUMOR

Glomus tumor

Localized multinucleate, distal, subungual keratosis[68]

Onychopapilloma of the nail bed[69,70]

Osteoma cutis in the nail matrix[71]

Idiopathic polydactylous longitudinal erythronychia[71]

LOCAL MALIGNANCY

Basal cell carcinoma[73]

Bowen's disease[69,74]

Malignant melanoma

Reproduced with permission from Baran R, Dawber RPR, de Berker DAR, Haneke E, Tosti A, eds. Baran and Dawber's Diseases of the Nails and their Management, 3rd edn. Oxford: Blackwell Science, 2001.

nail bed and the proliferation and fragility of these capillaries in active psoriasis. Splinter hemorrhages of the nail may be considered analogous to the Auspitz sign (bleeding point upon scraping) on the skin, but they occur in the nail bed. Splinter hemorrhages may be observed in psoriatic mimicry (Figure 6.38).

When initially formed, they are plum-colored, but darken to brown or black within days. The blood attaches itself to the underlying

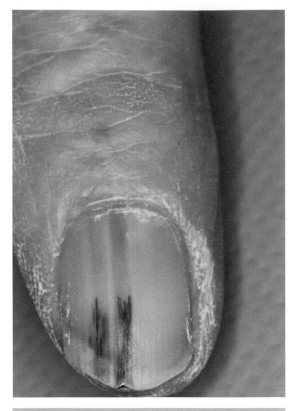

■ FIGURE 6.32

Idiopathic double longitudinal erythronychia associated with distal linear hemorrhages.

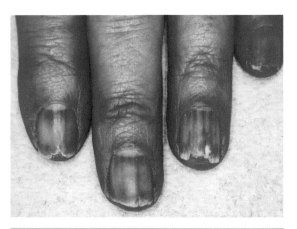

■ FIGURE 6.33

Idiopathic polydactylous longitudinal erythronychia. (Courtesy of B Krayen-Bühl, Switzerland and reproduced from Baran et al. Br J Dermatol 2006; 155: 219–21.)

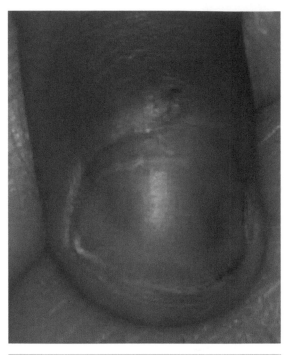

■ FIGURE 6.34

Hemangioma of the subungual tissues with pseudoclubbing. (Courtesy of BM Piraccini, Italy.)

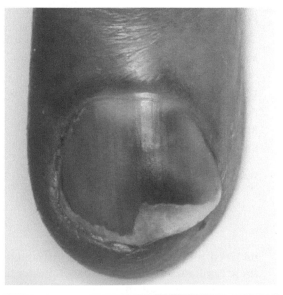

■ FIGURE 6.35

Glomus tumor of the nail bed.

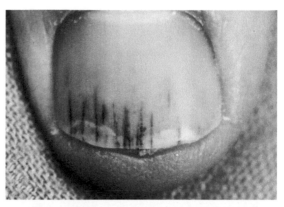

Splinter hemorrhages in psoriatic mimicry. (Courtesy of E Duhard, France.)

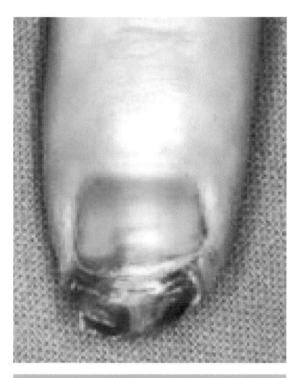

■ FIGURE 6.36

Angiolymphoid hyperplasia with eosinophilia. (Courtesy of JM Mascaro, Spain.)

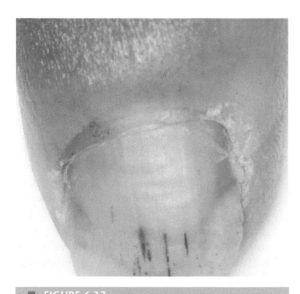

■ FIGURE 6.37

Psoriatic splinter hemorrhages.

nail plate and moves distally. Splinter hemorrhages occasionally appear to remain stationary, because of attachment to the nail bed rather than to the plate.[33]

The majority of splinter hemorrhages originate within the distal third of the nail, where the nail plate separates from the nail bed. In this region, especially delicate spirally wound capillaries produce the pink line normally seen through the nail about 4 mm proximal to the tip of the finger. Rupture of these superficially located thin-walled vessels gives rise to linear hemorrhages looking like wood splinters under the nails. Rare varieties of proximal splinter hemorrhages include onychomatricoma, Langerhans' cell histiocytosis, trichinosis, and mono- or polydactylous longitudinal erythronychia.

Splinter hemorrhages are more common in males than in females, and in dark-colored individuals than in whites. Age-associated nail changes and disorders are common in elderly patients, where splinter hemorrhages are the most common.

When present in females, they are typically confined to a single digit.

Trauma to the nail is prone to produce subungual hemorrhages, as are a number of drugs, including docetaxel, paclitaxel, and above all imatinib (Figure 6.39).

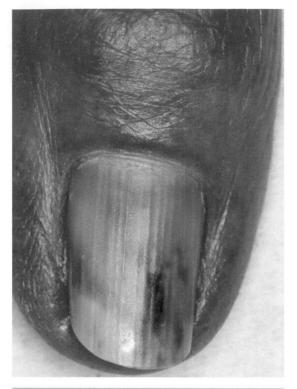

Splinter hemorrhages due to imatinib.

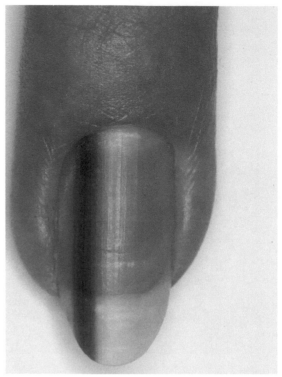

Longitudinal melanonychia following PUVA therapy.

Repeated microtrauma with partial overlapping of the second toe on the big toenail is responsible for bilateral triangular hemorrhages. Major causes of splinter hemorrhages are listed in Table 6.5.

■■■ NAIL MELANIN PIGMENTATION

PUVA therapy may activate melanocytes of the distal matrix and nail bed as longitudinal (Figure 6.40) and/or transverse melanonychia. Low-voltage X-ray are used (mainly in Switzerland and Germany) for treating nail psoriasis. Similar side-effects may be observed.

Nail melanin pigmentation should be distinguished from nonmelanin hyperchromia such as that due to topical drugs (e.g. the dark orange hue produced by anthralin; see page 3) and hematoma, especially that due to repeated minor trauma (friction from shoes, which may mimic a longitudinal streak).[34] However, the latter may be associated with foot deformities and/or unsatisfactory footwear in psoriatic patients.

Diagnosis of hematoma is usually easy, by applying a drop of immersion oil to the nail plate and using a strong magnifying lens or dermatoscope to show tiny globules of dried blood. A small disk of nail plate may be punched out after immersing the foot for 10 minutes in warm water, which renders the nail softer. The dark coloration is positive for blood with the pseudoperoxidase reaction (Hemostix test). Histopathology reveals lakes of blood that are peroxidase-positive but Prussian blue-negative.

■ TABLE 6.5

Major causes of splinter hemorrhages[33]

Skin diseases	Systemic diseases	Drugs	Others
Psoriasis	Subacute bacterial	Tetracycline	Trauma
Dermatitis/eczema	endocarditis	Oncohematological drugs	Idiopathic
Vasculitis	Fungal endocarditis	Drug reactions	Occupational hazards
Exfoliative dermatitis	Subacute lupus		Scurvy
Onychomycosis	erythematosus		Septicemia
Pterygium	Antiphospholipid syndrome		High-altitude living
Mycosis fungoides	Arterial emboli		Hemodialysis
Rendu–Osler–Weber syndrome	Hypertension		Peritoneal dialysis
Behçet's disease	Mitral stenosis		Indwelling brachial artery
Buerger's disease	Arthritis		cannula
Darier's disease	Trichinosis		Radial artery puncture
Histiocytosis X	Hypoparathyroidism		Severe illness
Collagen vascular disease	Diabetes mellitus		
Sweet syndrome	Peptic ulcer		
	Cirrhosis		
	Internal malignancy		
	Thyrotoxicosis		
	Raynaud's disease		
	Sarcoidosis		
	Hemochromatosis		
	Blood dyscrasias		
	Cryoglobulinemia		
	Renal disease		
	Pulmonary disease		
	Malignant neoplasia		

Reproduced with permission from Saladi et al. J Am Acad Dermatol 2004; 54: 289–92.

Nail melanin pigmentation is sometimes exogenous, due to fungal infection (*Trichophyton rubrum nigricans* or dematiaceous fungi, etc.). Such a melanonychia starts distal to proximal (Figure 6.41).

By contrast, nail melanin pigmentation as longitudinal melanonychia is produced by matrix focal melanocytic activation due to drugs (Figure 6.42), radiation, endocrine conditions, HIV infection, inflammatory nail disorders, Laugier's disease (Figure 6.43), Peutz–Jeghers syndrome, nonmelanocytic tumors (Figure 6.44), nutritional pigmentation, and traumatic origin (Figure 6.45). Matrix melanocytic pigmentation may also result in transverse melanonychia (due to cytotoxic drugs (Figure 6.46) or electron-beam therapy).[35]

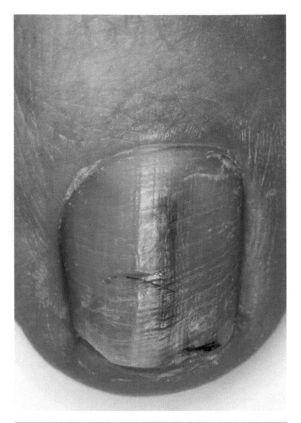

■ **FIGURE 6.41**

Longitudinal fungal melanonychia due to *Trichophyton rubrum*.

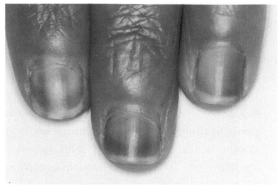

■ **FIGURE 6.42**

Melanonychia due to cytotoxic drugs.

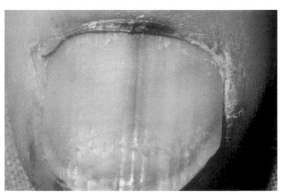

■ **FIGURE 6.43**

Laugier's disease: longitudinal melanonychia associated with pseudo Hutchinson's sign.

Nail pigmentation due to melanocytic proliferation should alert the physician when there is:

- any isolated pigmentation of a single digit during the fourth to sixth decade of life (melanoma can be seen in children, but is very rare)
- nail pigmentation that develops abruptly in a previously normal nail plate
- pigmentation that suddenly becomes darker, larger (Figure 6.47), or blurred (toward the nail matrix)
- acquired pigmentation of the thumb, index finger, or big toe
- a history of digital trauma

- recently acquired isolated pigmentation in a dark-skinned patient (particularly of the thumb or the big toe)
- any acquired lesion in a patient with a personal history of melanoma (Figure 6.48)
- pigmentation associated with nail dystrophy (partial nail destruction or absence of the nail plate)
- pigmentation of the periungual skin (Hutchinson's sign) (Figure 6.49), which should be differentiated from pseudo Hutchinson's sign (Figure 6.50)

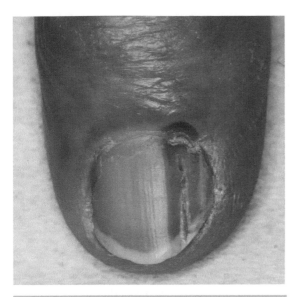

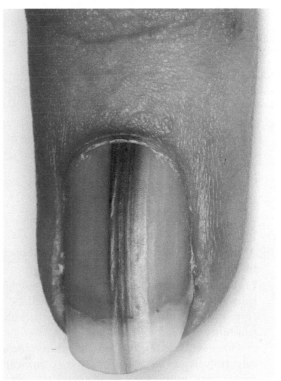

■ FIGURE 6.46

Combination of transverse and longitudinal melanonychia with transverse leukonychia.

■ FIGURE 6.44

Longitudinal melanonychia associated with myxoid pseudocyst.

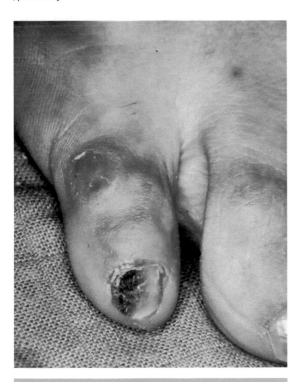

■ FIGURE 6.45

Frictional lateral melanonychia.

■ FIGURE 6.47

Proximal enlargement of longitudinal melanonychia (melanoma in situ).

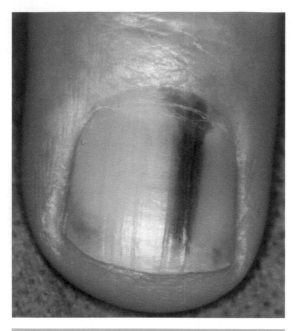

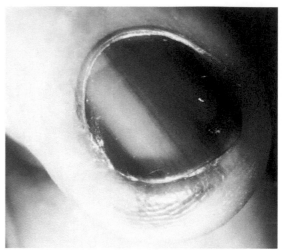

■ FIGURE 6.49

Melanonychia associated with Hutchison's sign

■ FIGURE 6.48

Metastasis of a melanoma of the back. (Courtesy of E Grosshans, France.)

Dermoscopy should be used systematically for the evaluation of nail pigmentation before deciding the necessity for a biopsy – which is indispensable when one is faced with any of the morphological changes listed above[36] (Figures 6.51 and 6.52).

■■■ GREEN NAILS

A yellow-green hue to the nail may be observed in psoriasis (Figure 6.53) due to the serum–like proteinaceous exudate, as well as in *Pseudomonas* infection. The latter should be excluded by culture, Wood's lamp examination, and chloroform solubility test.

However, contamination of paronychia and onycholysis by *Pseudomonas* is common in psoriasis (Figure 6.54).

Green nail syndrome[37] is characterized by a triad of green discoloration of the nail plate (Figure 6.55), paronychia, and *Pseudomonas* infection.

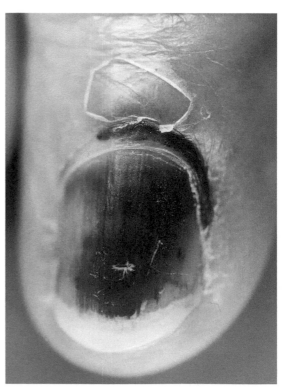

■ FIGURE 6.50

Subungual hematoma presenting as pseudo Hutchison's sign. (Courtesy of R Sinclair, Australia.)

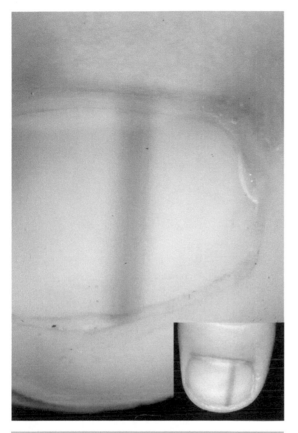

FIGURE 6.51

Dermoscopy of a longitudinal melanonychia due to a nevus in a child. (Courtesy of L Thomas, France.)

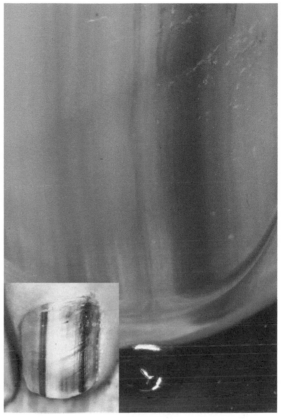

FIGURE 6.52

Dermoscopy of a melanoma in situ. (Courtesy of L Thomas, France.)

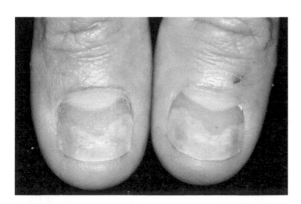

FIGURE 6.53

Yellow–green nails in psoriasis.

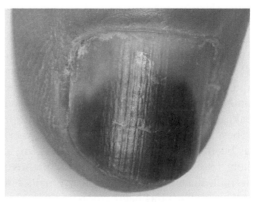

FIGURE 6.54

Pseudomonas infection (colonization of onycholysis in a psoriatic patient).

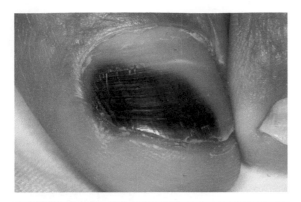

■ FIGURE 6.55

Pseudomonas infection in a jogger.

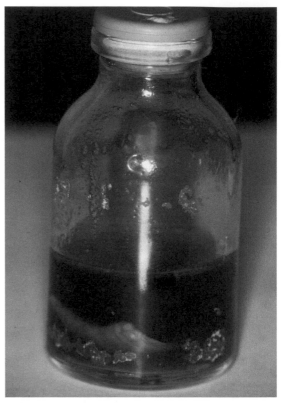

■ FIGURE 6.56

Chloroform test: the liquid turns green.

Pseudomonas spp. can colonize any area of the nail where there is onycholysis, as well as the nail fold. The pigmentation that follows this colonization varies both with the species involved and with the composition of the pigments produced. The colors vary correspondingly from a light green to a dark green/black. *Pseudomonas* spp. produce a number of different diffusible pigments, including pyocyanin (dark green) and fluorescein (yellow–green).[38–40] These are soluble in water, the former also in chloroform (Figure 6.56). This discoloration may involve the entire nail plate or simply part of it. Green-striped nails (Figure 6.57) may result from repeated episodes of bacterial infection in the proximal nail fold, with deposition of organisms and pigment during each episode. Some help in the diagnosis can be obtained by soaking nail fragments in water or chloroform. If these turn green, it is likely that *Pseudomonas* has been or is still present, and this is the most likely reason for the deposition of pigment in the nail. Black discoloration of the nails due to *Proteus mirabilis* has been reported.[41]

It is now no longer believed that *Candida* spp. or *Aspergillus* spp. are responsible for the green hue.

■■■ YELLOW NAILS

While psoriatic nails may present with a yellowish color (Figure 6.58), a yellow hue is also observed in onychomycosis, with distal to proximal longitudinal single or multiple streaks (Figure 6.59). More often, yellowish spots or patches appear irregular and haphazard.

The yellow nail syndrome is an uncommon disorder of unknown etiology characterized by the triad of yellow nails, lymphedema, and respiratory tract involvement. The entire nail plate shows a diffuse pale yellow to dark yellow–green discoloration (Figure 6.60). The edges of the nails are occasionally darker than the remainder, and the proximal part can sometimes maintain a

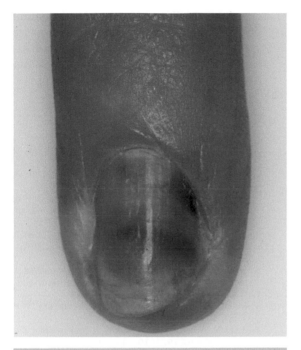

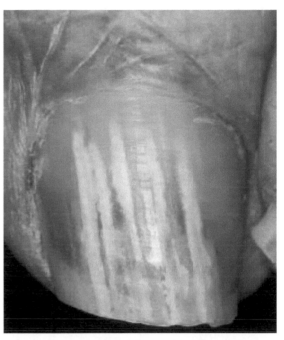

■ FIGURE 6.57

Transverse green-striped nail due to paronychial flares of *Pseudomonas* infection.

■ FIGURE 6.59

Yellow hue in multiple onychomycotic streaks.

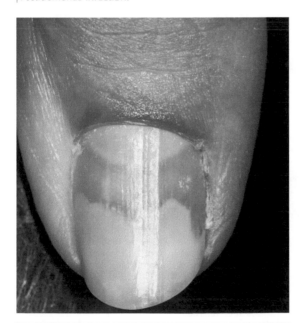

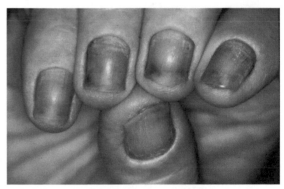

■ FIGURE 6.58

Psoriatic yellowish color in onycholysis.

■ FIGURE 6.60

Yellow nail syndrome.

normal color. The nails usually thickened and hardened demonstrate an increase in both transverse and longitudinal curvature. However, a marked decrease in the linear nail growth is probably a significant factor in causing nail dystrophy. Chronic paronychia can be seen.

Yellow nail syndrome has been reported in graft-versus-host disease (Figure 6.61).[42]

Lichen planus may mimic a yellow nail syndrome restricted to the digits[43–45] (Figure 6.62).

Onychomatricoma (see Chapter 10) presents with a longitudinal xanthonychia, usually involving one digit.

Several causes of nail discoloration may present with a golden nail color.

Chrysotherapy may produce, several months after the beginning of treatment, an orange-yellowish hue on all finger nails, as well as on the distal toenails. A yellow color may result from Divalproex sodium (Depakote®), pheny-

toin, lithium, fluorosis, carotinemia, jaundice. Tetracyclines may produce a yellow fluorescence of the lunulae under Wood's lamp and exceptionally a yellow discoloration in patients treated with these drugs for a long standing acne.

■■■ REFERENCES

1. Zaias N. Psoriasis of the nail. A clinical–pathology study. Arch Dermatol 1969; 99: 567–79.
2. Kates SL, Harris GD, Nagle DJ. Leukonychia totalis. J Hand Surg 1986; 11B, 465–6.
3. Albright SD, Wheeler CI. Leukonychia. Total and partial leukonychia in a single family with a review of the literature. Arch Dermatol 1964; 90: 392.
4. Baran R, Perrin C. Transverse leuconychia of toenail due to repeated microtrauma. Br J Dermatol, 1995; 133: 267–9.
5. Held JL, Chew S, Grossman ME, et al. Transverse striate leukonychia associated with rejection of renal allograft. J Am Acad Dermatol 1989; 20: 513–14.
6. Mitchell JC. A clinical study of leukonychia. Br J Dermatol 1953; 65: 121–30.
7. Zaias N, Ackerman AB. The nail in Darier–White disease. Arch Dermatol 1973; 107: 193–9.
8. Moulin G, Baran R, Perrin Ch. Epidermal hamartoma presenting as longitudinal pachyleukonychia: a new nail genodermatosis. J Am Acad Dermatol 1996; 35: 675–7.
9. Terry RB. White nails in hepatic cirrhosis. Lancet 1954; i: 757.
10. Holzberg M, Walker HK. Terry's nails : revised definition and new correlations. Lancet 1984; i: 896–9.
11. Lindsay PG. The half-and-half nail. Arch Intern Med 1967; 119: 583.
12. Daniel CR, Bower JD, Daniel CR Jr. The half-and-half fingernail. The most significant onychopathological indicator of chronic renal failure. J Miss St Med Assoc 1975; 16: 367–70.
13. Nixon DW, Pirrozi D, York RM, et al. Dermatologic changes after systemic cancer therapy. Cutis 1981; 27: 181.
14. Muehrcke RC. The fingernails in chronic hypoalbuminemia. BMJ 1956; i: 1327
15. Feldman SR, Gammon WR. Unilateral Muehrcke's lines following trauma. Arch Dermatol 1989; 125: 133–4.
16. Horan MA, Puxty JA, Fox RA. The white nails of old age (Neapolitan nails). J Am Geriatr Soc 1982; 30: 734–7.
17. Brauer E, Baran R. Cosmetics: the care and adornment of the nail. In: Baran R, Dawber RPR, De Berker D, Haneke E, Tosti A, eds. Baran and Dawber's Nail Diseases and Their Management, 3rd edn. Oxford: Blackwell Science, 2001. pp 358–69.
18. Ena P, Mazzarello V, Fenu G, Rubino C. Leukonychia from 2-ethyl-cyanoacrylate glue. Contact Dermatitis 2000; 42: 105.
19. Runne U, Organos CE. The human nail: structure, growth and pathological changes. Curr Probl Dermatol 1981; 9: 102–49.

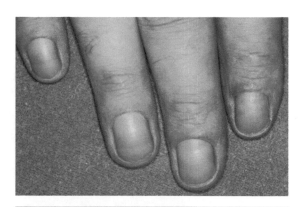

■ FIGURE 6.61

Graft-versus-host disease presenting as yellow nail syndrome. (Courtesy of JM Mascaró, Spain.)

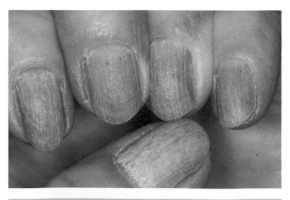

■ FIGURE 6.62

Lichen planus mimicking yellow nail syndrome.

20. Eichmann A, Baran R. Lectitis purulenta et granulomatosa. Dermatology 1998; 196: 352–3.

21. Shelley WB. The spotted lunula. J Am Acad Dermatol 1980; 2: 385–7.

22. Bergner T, Donhauser G, Ruzicka T. Red lunulae in alopecia areata. Acta Derma Venereol 1992; 72: 203–5.

23. Terry R. Red half-moon in cardiac failure. Lancet 1954; ii: 842–4.

24. De Berker DAR, Perrin C, Baran R. Localized longitudinal erythronychia. Diagnostic significance and physical explanation. Arch Dermatol 2004; 140: 1253–7.

25. Baran R, Perrin Ch. Longitudinal erythronychia with distal subungual keratosis: Onychopapilloma of the nail bed and Bowen's disease. Br J Dermatol 2000; 143: 132–5.

26. Piraccini BM, Antonucci A, Rech G et al. Congenital pseudoclubbing of a finger nail caused by subungual hemangioma. J Am Acad Dermatol 2005; 53: S123–6.

27. Burge SM, Baran R, Dawber RPR, et al. Periungual and arteriovenous tumours. Br J Dermatol 1986; 115: 361–6.

28. Cornill C, Toscas I, Mascaro JM, et al. Angiolymphoid hyperplasia with eosinophilia of the nail bed and bone: successful treatment with radiation therapy. J Eur Acad Dermatol Venereol 2004; 18: 584–5.

29. Graft GE. A review of hereditary hemorrhagic telangiectasia. J Am Osteo Assoc 1983; 82: 412.

30. Viseux V, Boulenger A, Jestin B, Plantin P. Transient subungual erythema in a patient with idiopathic Sweet's syndrome. J Am Acad Dermatol 2003; 49: 554–5.

31. Calvert HT, Smith MA, Wells RS. Psoriasis and the nails. Br J Dermatol 1963; 75: 415.

32. Scher RK, Daniel R. Nails: Therapy, Diagnosis, Surgery. Philadelphia: WB Saunders, 1990.

33. Saladi RN, Persaud AN, Rudikoff D, Cohen SR. Idiopathic splinter hemorrhages. J Am Acad Dermatol 2004; 50: 289–92.

34. Baran R, Perrin C, Thomas L, Braun R. The melanocytic system of the nail and its disorders. In: Nordlund JJ, Boissy RE, Hearing J et al, eds. The Pigmentary System. Oxford: Blackwell Science, 2006: 1037–48.

35. Quinlan KE, Janiga JJ, Baran R, et al. Transverse melanonychia secondary to total skin electron beam therapy: a report of 3 cases. J Am Acad Dermatol 2005; 53(2 Suppl 1): S112–14.

36. Ronger S, Touzet S, Ligeron C, et al. Dermoscopic examination of nail pigmentation. Arch Dermatol 2002; 138: 1327–33.

37. Goldman L, Fox H. Greenish pigmentation of nail plates from Bacillus pyocyaneus infection. Arch Derm Syph 1944; 49: 136–57.

38. Bauer MF, Cohen BA. The role of Pseudomonas in infection about the nails. Arch Dermatol 1957; 75: 394–6

39. Moore M, Marcus MD. Green nails. Role of Candida and Pseudomonas aeruginosa. Arch Dermatol 1951; 64: 499–505

40. Chernosky M, Dukes D. Green nails. Arch Dermatol 1963; 88: 548–553

41. Qadripur SA, Schauder S, Schwartz P. Black nails from Proteus mirabilis colonisation. Hautarzt 2001; 52: 658–61.

42. Mascaró JM, Martin-Ortega. Nail alterations in GVHD. In: Dermatology Progress and Perspectives. New York. Parthenon: 1993; 393–4.

43. Haneke E. Isolated bullous lichen planus of the nails mimicking yellow nail syndrome. Clin Exp Dermatol 1983; 8: 425–8.

44. Tosti A, Piraccini BM, Cameli N. Nail changes in lichen planus may resemble those of yellow nail syndrome. Br J Dermatol 2000; 142: 848–9.

45. Baran R. Lichen planus of the nails mimicking the yellow nail syndrome. Br J Dermatol 2000; 143: 1117–18.

46. McGrae JD. Keratitis, ichthyosis and deafness (KID) syndrome. Int J Dermatol 1990; 29: 89.

47. Huriez CL, Deminati M, Agache P et al. Génodermatose scléro-atrophiante et kératodermique des extrémités. Ann Dermatol Vénéréol 1969; 6: 135.

48. Voron DA, Hatfield HH, Kalkhoff RX. Multiple lentigines syndrome. Case report and review of literature. Am J Med 1976; 60: 446.

49. Stevens KR, Leis PF, Peters S et al. Congenital leukonychia. J Am Acad Dermatol 1998; 39: 509.

50. Yamamoto T, Tohyama J, Koeda T et al. Multiple epiphyseal dysplasia with small head, congenital nystagmus, hypoplasia of corpus callosum, and leukonychia totalis: a variant of Lowry–Wood syndrome? Am J Med Genet. 1995; 56: 6–9.

51. Mahler RH, Gerstein W, Watters K. Congenital leukonychia striata. Cutis 1987; 39: 453–4.

52. Baran R, Achten G. Les associations congénitales de koïlonychie et de leuconychie totale. Arch Belges Dermatol 1969; 25: 13–29.

53. Crosti C, Sala F, Bertani E et al. Leukonychia totalis and ectodermal dysplasia: report of 2 cases. Ann Dermatol Venereol 1983; 110: 617–22.

54. Buskshell LL, Gorlin AJ. Leukonychia totalis, multiple subaceous cysts, renal calculi. Arch Dermatol 1975; 111: 899.

55. Friedel J, Heid E, Grosshans E. Le syndrome FLOTCH: survenue familiale d'une leuconychie totale, de kystes trichilemmaux et d'une dystrophie ciliaire, à hérédité autosomique dominante. Ann Dermatol Venereol 1986; 113: 549.

56. Moshkowitz A, Abrahamov A, Pisani S. Congenital hypoparathyroidism simultating epilepsy, with other symptoms and dental signs of intra-uterine hypocalcemia. Pediatrics 1969; 44: 401.

57. Ingegno AP, Yatto RP. Hereditary white nails (leukonychia totalis), duodenal ulcer, and gallstones. Genetic implications of a syndrome. NY State J Med 1982; 82: 1797–800.

58. Giustina TA, Woo TX, Campbell JP et al. Association of pili torti and leukonychia. Cutis 1985; 35: 573.

59. Schueller WA. Acrokeratosis verruciformis of Hopf. Arch Dermatol 1972; 106: 81.

60. Hoffman MD, Flemming MG, Pearson RW. Acantholytic epidermolysis bullosa. Arch Dermatol 1995; 131: 586–9.

61. Venencie PY, Dallot A. Acantholytic dyskeratotic epidermal nevus: a mosaic form of Darier's disease? Ann Dermatol Venereol 1997; 126: 829–30.

62. Higashi N. Focal acantholytic dyskeratosis. Hifu 1990; 32: 507–10.

63. Baran R, Perrin C. Focal subungal warty dyskeratoma. Dermatology 1997; 195: 77–82.
64. McLean TK, Lane JE, Scher R, Lesher JL. Bilobed thumbnails with erythronychia. J Cutan Med Surg 2003; 7: 458–9.
65. Lesher JL Jr, Peterson CM, Lane JE. An unusual case of factitious onychodystrophy Pediatr Dermatol. 2004; 21: 272–3.
66. Siragusa M, Schepis C, Consentino F et al. Nail pathology in patients with hemiplegia. Br J Dermatol 2001; 144: 557–60.
67. Siragusa M, Del Graco S, Ferri R et al. Longitudinal red streaks on the big toenails in a patient with pseudo-bulbar syndrome. JEADV 2001; 15: 77–92.
68. Baran R, Perrin C. Localized multinucleate distal subungual keratosis. Br J Dermatol 1995; 133: 77–82.
69. Baran R, Perrin C. Longitudinal erythronychia with distal subungual keratosis: onychopapilloma of the nail bed and Bowen's disease. Br J Dermatol 2000; 143: 132–5.
70. De Berker DA, Perrin C, Baran R. Localized longitudinal erythronychia. Diagnostic significance and physical explanation. Arch Dermatol 2004; 140: 1253–7.
71. Blatière V, Baran R, Barnéon G. An osteoma cutis of the nail matrix. JEADV 1999; 12(suppl 25): 126.
72. Baran R, Dawber RPR, Perrin C. Idiopathic polydactylous longitudinal erythronychia: a newly described entity. Br J Dermatol 2006; 155: 219–21.
73. Gee BC, Millard PR, Dawber RPR. Onychopapilloma is not a distinct clinico-pathological entity. Br J Dermatol 2002; 146: 156–7.
74. Reuter G, Keller F, Samama F et al. Maladie de Bowen unguéale à type d'érythronychie. Aspect dermoscopique et étude virologique. Ann Dermatol Vénéréol 2005; 132: 596–614.

Chapter 7

Acro-osteolysis

Approximately 7% of patients with psoriasis have arthritis and 3–5% of patients with chronic polyarthritis have psoriasis,[1] while nail changes have been noted in 86.5% of patients affected by arthropathic psoriasis[2] (Figure 7.1).

Less than 15% of peripheral forms of psoriatic rheumatism present with acro-osteolysis, mostly as the longitudinal type, associated with distal interphalangeal arthritis. Interestingly, proximal interphalangeal and metatarsal digital joints may also be affected. The defect is more frequent in toes than in fingers. Exceptionally, acro-osteolysis may appear without joint involvement.[3,4]

Psoriasis and arthritis may occur together coincidentally or as associated lesions.

- When psoriasis accompanies otherwise classic rheumatoid arthritis, the majority of patients have positive tests for rheumatoid factor.
- When the arthritis is not classically rheumatoid, there is a predilection for involvement of the terminal interphalangeal joints[2] (Figure 7.2).

The arthritis associated with psoriasis is generally milder with fewer joints being affected than in normal cases of rheumatoid arthritis, but it may be more destructive and erosive of the bone and may produce arthritis mutilans. This is found in less than 5% of patients with psoriasis and arthritis, usually involving the hands and feet. It

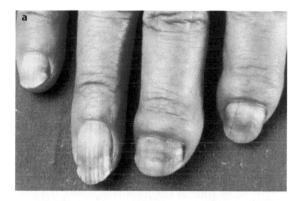

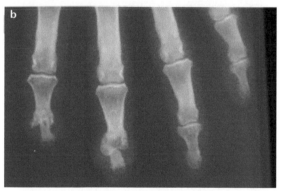

■ FIGURE 7.1

(a) Arthropathic psoriasis with acro-osteolysis. (b) The same patient presenting with osteolysis. (Part (a) courtesy of P Combemale, France.)

is characteristically an asymmetric osteolytic arthropathy that begins at the articular surfaces and destroys the joint. Juxta-articular bone resorption results in shortening of the digits,

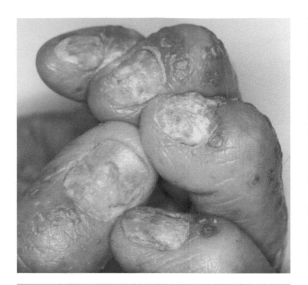

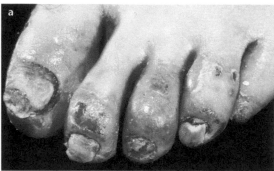

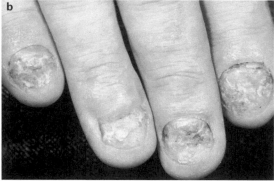

■ **FIGURE 7.2**

Psoriatic arthritis with involvement of the terminal interphalangeal joints.

with telescoping of the proximal and distal ends of the joints (opera-glass hand).[5]

The psoriasis sometimes appears after or at the same time as the joint symptoms, but usually it precedes the arthritis.

X-rays show joint widening and destruction of subchondral bone as in rheumatoid arthritis, and these features also appear in the distal interphalangeal joints, with simultaneous erosion of the terminal phalanges. The cystic changes and the irregularities of the tufts of the distal phalanges progressing to whittling away of the bone to become peg-shaped, which is very characteristic of psoriatic arthritis. Osteolysis itself is characteristic of psoriasis, and may be a precursor of gross destruction.

Pustular psoriasis and acrodermatitis continua suppurativa (Hallopeau) are classical conditions likely to induce merely longitudinal acro-osteolysis[6] (Figure 7.3).

It has been suggested that the bone lesions may represent a 'deep Koebner effect'.[7]

Distal phalangeal tuft resorption, in the absence of severe proximal joint destruction, has been reported in severe pustular psoriasis.

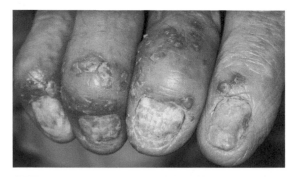

■ FIGURE 7.3(a,b)

Acrodermatitis continua suppurativa. (Part (a) courtesy of A Griffiths, UK.)

■ **FIGURE 7.4**

Psoriatic arthritis resembling gout.

Diagnosis of psoriatic arthritis can be challenging because of signs and symptoms in common with other arthropathies, including rheumatoid arthritis, osteoarthritis, and gout (Figure 7.4).

The term acro-osteolysis denotes the occurrence of destructive changes of the distal phalangeal bone. Shortening of the distal phalanges causes the nails to appear abnormally broad (acquired racket-shaped digits)[8] (Figure 7.5). The cutaneous signs of acro-osteolysis range from bulbous fingertips with soft tissue thickening associated with pseudoclubbing (Figure 7.6a)

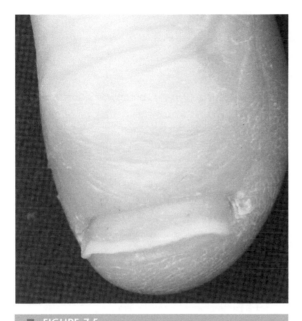

■ FIGURE 7.5

Acquired racket-shaped digit. (Courtesy of B Schubert, France.)

(defined as an overcurvature of the nails in both the longitudinal and transverse axes, with preservation of a normal Lovibond angle) to severe destruction of the digits and metacarpal or metatarsal bones.[9] Koilonychia may be observed.[10] Pincer nail deformity has occurred after traumatic acro-osteolysis. In severe cases, the nail unit can be destroyed. Deformation and destruction of the digits is commonly accompanied by trophic changes in soft tissues and ulcerations.[11,12]

Functional symptoms such as acroparesthesia, dull pain, or vasospastic changes of the digits (Figure 7.7) can be early manifestations of acro-osteolysis. Acro-osteolysis can be idiopathic (familial or nonfamilial) or it can occur in association with a number of metabolic (Figure 7.8), neuropathic (Figures 7.9 and 7.10), and collagen (Figures 7.11 and 7.12) disorders (Table 7.1).

In familial acro-osteolysis, pain is a conspicuous symptom. On radiographic examination, two varieties of acro-osteolysis may occur together or independently: transverse acro-osteolysis (Figures 7.13, 7.14a,b) and longitudinal acro-osteolysis.[13,14] In transverse acro-osteolysis, the distal phalangeal shaft shows a transverse lytic band, while the tuft and base are preserved. Fragmentation of the separated distal tuft can occur with near total loss of the tuft, i.e. acronecrosis (Figure 7.12b). In longitudinal acro-osteolysis (Figure 7.15), terminal resorption of the distal end of the phalanx progressively results in a 'licked candystick'

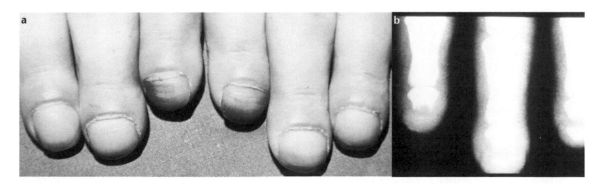

■ FIGURE 7.6

(a) Pseudoclubbing in vinyl chloride disease. (b) X-rays showing transverse acro-osteolysis. (Courtesy of G Moulin, France.)

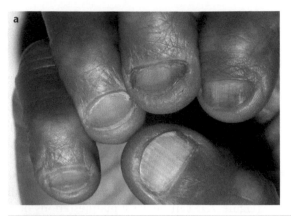

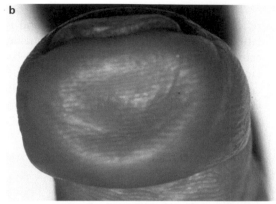

■ FIGURE 7.7

(a) Raynaud's disease. (b) The same patient showing distal pulp depression. (Part (a) courtesy of S Goettmann-Bonvallot, France.)

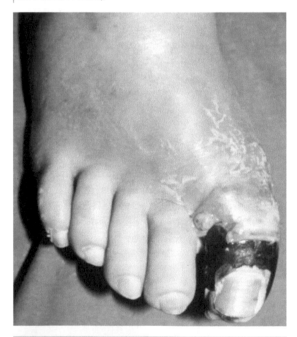

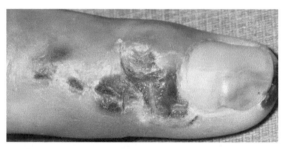

■ FIGURE 7.9

Carpal canal syndrome with acro-osteolysis. (Courtesy of F Lemarchand-Venencie, France.)

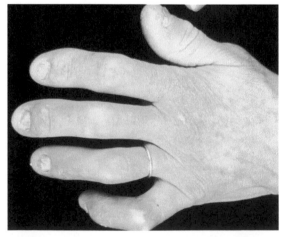

■ FIGURE 7.8

Diabetic gangrene. (Courtesy of A Raganelli, Italy.)

appearance of phalangeal, metacarpal, or meta-tarsal bones. The transverse radiological pattern is characteristic of vinyl chloride disease[15] (Figure 7.6), renal osteodystrophy (Figure 7.16), idiopathic nonfamilial acro-osteolysis, and familial acro-osteolysis. In longitudinal acro-osteolysis,

■ FIGURE 7.10

Syringomyelia.

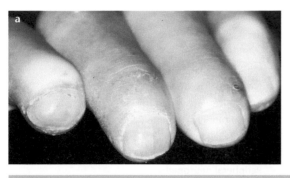

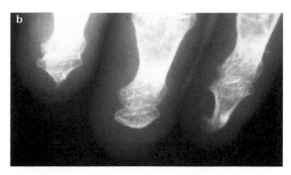

■ FIGURE 7.11

(a) Scleroderma with finger involvement. (b) The same patient with acronecrosis.

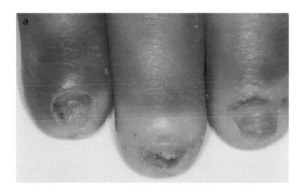

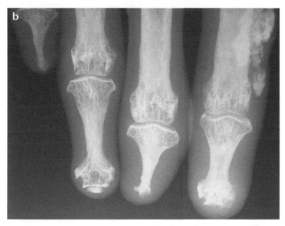

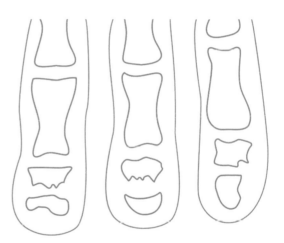

■ FIGURE 7.13

Transverse acro-osteolysis, showing lytic bands. (After X Phelip and P Pras.)

which may be observed in scleroderma (Figures 7.11 and 7.12), hyperparathyroidism (Figure 7.5), chronic hemodialysis, psoriasis, neurological disorders[16] (Figures 7.9 and 7.10), frostbite (Figure 7.17), and bacterial infection[17] (Figures 7.18 and 7.19), cystic changes and irregularity of the distal tufts can be followed by severe bone resorption, resulting in pencilling of the phalanges. Progressive destruction of the bone produces peg-shaped phalanges.

■ FIGURE 7.12

(a) Acrosclerosis. (b) The same patient with peg-shaped phalanges.

Causes of acro-osteolysis

IDIOPATHIC ACRO-OSTEOLYSIS	Syringomyelia (Figure 7.10)
	Thromboangiitis obliterans
PRIMARY ACRO-OSTEOLYSIS	**Neuropathic diseases**
Ehlers–Danlos syndrome	Bureau–Barrière syndrome (see Chapter 10)
Familial mandibuloacral dysplasia	Carpal tunnel syndrome (Figure 7.9)
Hadju–Cheney syndrome	Congenital insensitivity to pain syndrome
Pachydermoperiostosis	Leprosy (Figures 7.14, 7.18, and 7.19)
Progeria	Peripheral neuropathy
Pyknodysostosis	Self-mutilation after spinal cord injury
Rothmund syndrome	Tabes dorsalis
Van Bogaert–Hazary syndrome	Thévenard syndrome
Werner syndrome	**Dermatological conditions**
	Acrodermatitis continua Hallopeau
ACQUIRED ACRO-OSTEOLYSIS	Epidermolysis bullosa
Arthropathies and collagen diseases	Ichthyosiform erythroderma
CREST syndrome	Juvenile hyaline fibromatosis
Farber's disease (Figure 7.20)	Mucopolysaccharidosis
Juvenile chronic arthritis	Pityriasis rubra pilaris
Mixed connective tissue disease	Porphyria cutanea tarda
Multicentric reticulohistiocytosis	Sézary syndrome
Osteoarthritis	**Physical injuries**
Polymyositis	Burns
Psoriasis	Frostbite (Figure 7.17)
Reiter syndrome	Fulguration
Rheumatoid arthritis	Mechanical stress (guitar players, Figure 7.22)
Sarcoidosis	**Toxic exposure**
Scleroderma	Polyvinyl chloride (Figure 7.6a,b)
Sjögren syndrome	Trichloroethylene
Systemic lupus erythematosus	Phenytoin
Metabolic and endocrine diseases	Ergot
Acromegaly	**Miscellaneous**
Diabetes mellitus	Adjuvant (Freund)
Gout	Distal phalanx infection
Hyperparathyroidism	Distal phalanx tumor:
Osteomalacia	Benign or malignant
Porphyria	Primary or metastatic
Renal osteodystrophy	Nutritional deficiencies
Vascular diseases	Snake or scorpion venom
Ainhum (Figure 7.21)	
Atherosclerosis	
Raynaud syndrome/disease (Figure 7.7a,b)	

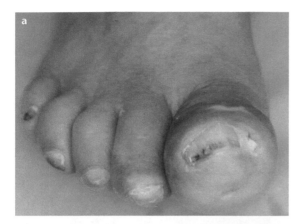

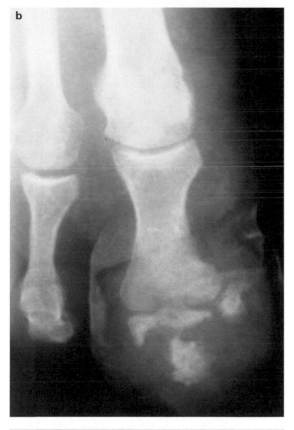

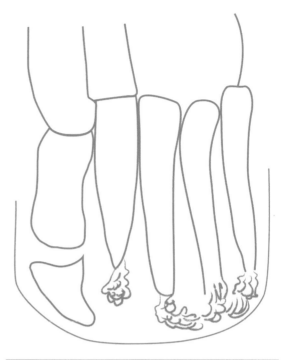

■ FIGURE 7.15

Longitudinal acro-osteolysis bands. (After X Phelip and P Pras.)

■ FIGURE 7.14

(a) Leprosy with abnormality of the big toe. (b) The same patient, showing acronecrosis. (Reproduced from Baran and Dawber. Diseases of the Nails, 3rd ed. Oxford: Blackwell Science, 2001, with kind permission of Blackwell Science.)

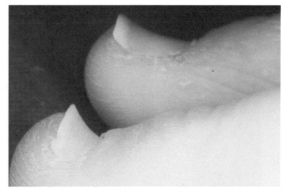

■ FIGURE 7.16

Renal osteodystrophy with shortening of the distal phalanges due to acro-osteolysis. (Courtesy of B Schubert, France.)

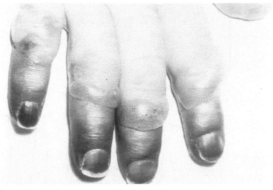

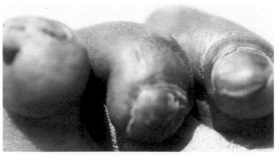

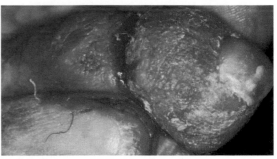

■ FIGURE 7.17

Frostbite. (Courtesy of E Webster, USA.)

■ FIGURE 7.18

Leprosy, with destruction of the distal phalanges.

■ FIGURE 7.19

Acronecrosis in leprosy. (Courtesy of P Queneau, France.)

■ FIGURE 7.21

Ainhum. (Courtesy of JJ Morand, France.)

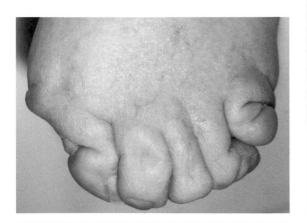

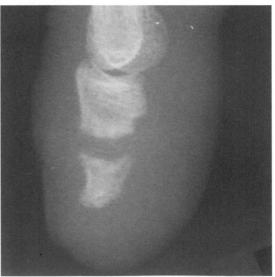

■ FIGURE 7.20

Arthropathy with acro-osteolysis in lipogranulomatosis of Farber. (Courtesy of JF Stalder, France.)

■ FIGURE 7.22

Acro-osteolysis in a guitar player. (Courtesy of JM Destouet and WA Murphy, USA.)

■■■ **REFERENCES**

1. Moll JMH, Wright V. Psoriasis arthritis. Semin Arthritis Rheum 1973; 3: 55–78.
2. Lavaroni G, Kokelj F, Paulouzzi P, et al. The nails in psoriatic arthritis. Acta Derma Venereol 1994; 186 (Suppl): 113.
3. Miller JL, Soltani K, Tourtellotte CD. Psoriatic acro-osteolysis without arthritis. J Bone Joint Surg 1971; 53: 371–4.
4. Cheesbrough MJ. Osteolysis and psoriasis. Clin Exp Dermatol 1979; 4: 341–4.
5. Mahowald ML, Parrish RM. Severe osteolytic arthritis mutilans in pustular psoriasis. Arch Dermatol 1982; 118: 434–7.
6. Combemale P, Baran R, Flechaire A, et al. Psoriatic acro-osteolysis. Exclusive subungual pustular form associated with distant psoriasis vulgaris. Ann Dermatol Venereol 1989; 116: 555–8.
7. Buckley WR, Raleigh RL. Psoriasis with acroosteolysis. N Engl J Med 1959; 261: 539–41.
8. Fairris GM, Rowell NR. Acquired racket nails. Clin Exp Dermatol 1984; 9: 267–9.
9. Meyerson LB, Meier GC. Cutaneous lesions in acro-osteolysis. Arch Dermatol 1972; 106: 224–7.
10. Nguyen V, Buk PL, Roberts B, et al. Koilonychia, dome-shaped epiphyses and vertebral platyspondylia. J Pediatr 2005; 147: 112–14.
11. Phelip X, Pras P. Les acro-ostéolyses. Rhumatologie 1975; 27: 325–33.
12. Queneau P, Gabbai A, Perpoint B, et al. Acro-ostéolyses au cours de la lèpre. Rev Rhum Mal Osteoartic 1982; 49: 111–19.
13. Destouet JM, Murphy WA. Acquired acroosteolysis and acronecrosis. Arthritis Rheum 1983; 26: 1150–4.
14. Kemp SS, Dalinka MK, Schumacher HR. Acro-osteolysis. Etiologic and radiological considerations. JAMA 1986; 255: 2058–61.
15. Markovitz SS, McDonald CJ, Fethiere W, et al. Occupational acrosteolysis. Arch Dermatol 1972; 106: 219–23.
16. Vanhooteghem O, Lateur N, Hautecoeur P, et al. Acropathia ulcero-mutilans acquisata of the upper limbs. Br J Dermatol 1999; 140: 334–7.
17. Pereira O, Velho GC, Lopes V, et al. Acral necrosis by *Stenotrophomonas maltophilia.* J Eur Acad Dermatol Venereol 2001; 15: 334–6.

Chapter 8

Dual pathology: onychomycosis and psoriasis

Psoriasis is the dermatosis that most frequently affects the nail, and onychomycosis is by far the most common nail disease. It is therefore not uncommon to have ungual psoriasis and a fungal nail infection at the same time (Figures 8.1 and 8.2).

A number of publications suggest that psoriasis appears to render a nail more susceptible to mycotic infection, particularly the toenails[1-8] (Table 8.1). These two conditions may look very similar, and in fact can also occur together: the same nail may have psoriasis

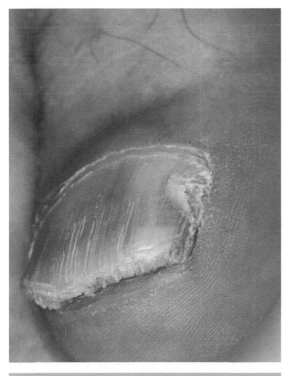

■ FIGURE 8.1

Psoriatic subungual hyperkeratosis associated with *Trichophyton rubrum* invasion.

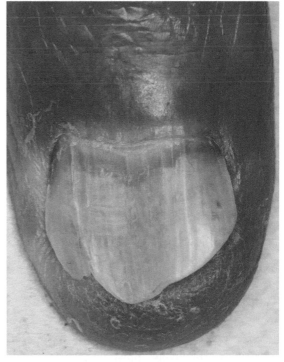

■ FIGURE 8.2

Psoriatic onycholysis associated with *Trichophyton rubrum* invasion.

Prevalence of onychomycosis in psoriasis

No. of psoriatics examined	Onychomycosis	Ref
100	14% dermatophytes	1
	16% *Candida* spp.	
	16% molds	
120	35% all fungi	2
	24% dermatophytes	
	15% *Candida albicans*	
78	27% all nail in psoriatics	3
	23% normal nails	
	30% altered nails	
561	13% all nails	7
	0.7% normal appearing nails	
	27% clinically abnormal nails	

and onychomycosis, or one nail may be psoriatic and a neighboring one onychomycotic. Histopathology and mycological culture may be the only means to differentiate these two conditions or prove that one nail suffers from both of them. Some differential diagnostic criteria may help to make the correct diagnosis.

There has been a generally held opinion that onychomycosis should be less frequent in psoriatic nails because dermatophytes do not survive in parakeratotic keratin and, in particular, are not found where there is pronounced exudation of serum, and hence serum inclusion in the parakeratosis. However, this is not the case, as many investigations, including some with deep nail biopsies, have shown.[9–12]

A correct diagnosis is essential for several reasons:

- to achieve successful treatment
- to explain the natural course of the disease
- to explain the therapeutic response
- to effectively prevent recurrences once treatment has been successful

Psoriatic nail changes are seen in approximately 7–13% of psoriatic children, in 50% of psoriasis patients at any given time, and in 80–90% during their lifetime.

Some of the features that psoriasis and onychomycosis have in common, as well as those distinguishing the two most important nail disorders, are listed in Table 8.2.[13–17] Further details are given below.

Onycholysis is very frequent in both psoriasis and onychomycosis. Whereas its proximal border is lined by a reddish-brown band in psoriasis, this is lacking in onychomycosis and other conditions characterized by onycholysis. It represents the active psoriatic lesion and is hence identical with the changes of a salmon spot. Onycholysis is also often due to trauma, cosmetic, infections, prolonged immersion in water, salt and sugar solutions, detergents and organic solvents, iron deficiency, atopic eczema, allergic and irritant contact dermatitis, vesicular skin diseases, erythema multiforme, Stevens–Johnson syndrome, toxic epidermal necrolysis, many drugs, and photo-onycholysis. Any of these

■ TABLE 8.2

Clinical features of psoriasis and onychomycosis

Clinical sign	Psoriasis	Onychomycosis
Frequency	1–2% of population affected	Increasing with age: 0.2% in children, >40% in elderly persons
Course	Chronic, remitting	Chronic, progressive
Symptoms	Usually none, cosmetic embarrassment	May be painful due to subungual hyperkeratosis, cosmetic embarrassment
Trauma	May induce lesions (Köbner phenomenon)	Predisposes to fungal infection
Pitting	Very frequent	Rare
Onycholysis	Frequent	Frequent
Discoloration[a]	None to yellow	None to yellow to brown
Salmon spots	Frequent	Very rare
Subungual hyperkeratosis	Frequent	Frequent
Nail plate thickening	Rare	Rare
Nail splitting	Rare	Frequent
Nail plate destruction	Particularly in arthropathic psoriasis	Always in total dystrophic onychomycosis
Splinter hemorrhage	Rare	None
Leukonychia	Rare, transverse	Mycotic leukonychia in superficial white onychomycosis
Paronychia	Rare	Rare in dermatophytoses, frequent in mold onychomycoses
Spores and hyphae	Rare	Very frequent
Transverse ridges	Rare	Rare
Genetic component	Particularly in type 1 psoriasis	Susceptibility to develop *Trychophyton rubrum*) onychomycosis is thought to be an autosomal dominant trait
Skin lesions elsewhere	Psoriasis elsewhere	Tinea pedum and/or manuum, tinea corporis

[a]Bacterial colonization and exogenous substances may modify the color of the nail.

conditions can occur in association with psoriasis or onychomycosis.

Subungual hyperkeratosis is also frequent in both psoriasis and onychomycosis. It contains large amounts of parakeratosis, usually in a layered arrangement, in psoriasis. Neutrophils may be compressed between the parakeratotic lamellae, forming Munro's abscesses (Figure 8.3). Small periodic acid–Schiff (PAS)-positive serum inclusions may also be present, and may resemble fungal elements. In psoriasis, the nail plate is usually rough, opaque, and lusterless. In onychomycosis, the subungual keratosis is mainly orthokeratotic, with a few parakeratotic areas intermingled. There are usually abundant hyphae, very often with spores. They are PAS-positive and found at the undersurface of the nail plate in distal subungual onychomycosis (Figures 8.4, 8.5 and 8.6) or within the entire nail plate in proximal subungual onychomycosis. But, in contrast to the small serum inclusions, their cell walls are more strongly PAS-positive. Intracorneal microabscesses are very frequently found. Subungual hyperkeratosis is also frequently due to chronic repeated trauma, chronic eczema, pityriasis rubra pilaris, overcurvature of the nail plate, lichen planus of the nail bed, erythroderma, acrokeratosis paraneoplastica, crusted scabies, dyskeratosis follicularis of Darier, and pachyonychia congenita (where it is extremely marked).

Table 8.3 shows the relationship between psoriasis and onychomycosis.

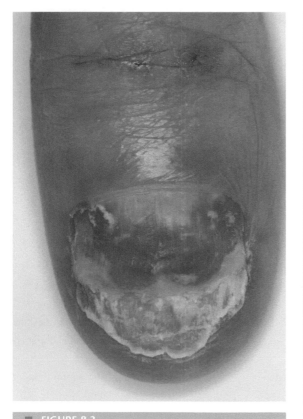

■ FIGURE 8.3

Pustular psoriasis associated with numerous hyphae invading the ventral nail plate histologically.

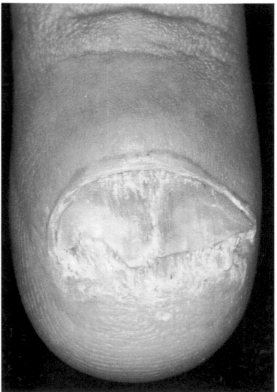

■ FIGURE 8.4

Candida infection in psoriatic distal subungual hyperkeratosis.

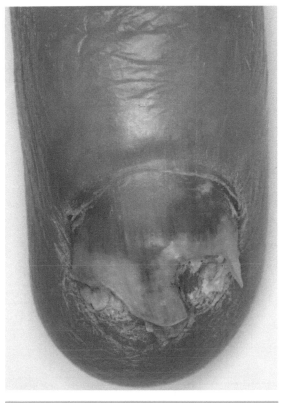

■ FIGURE 8.5

Psoriatic distal subungual hyperkeratosis associated with *Fusarium* spp.

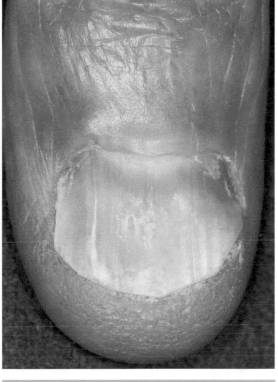

■ FIGURE 8.6

Psoriatic onycholysis associated with *Trichophyton rubrum* invasion.

■ TABLE 8.3

Relationship between psoriasis and onychomycosis

Heredity

Psoriasis
Mycotic colonization of a psoriatic nail
Onychomycotization of psoriasis
Induction of psoriasis by onychomycosis
(Köbner phenomenon)
Psoriasis and onychomycosis
Onychomycosis

Infection
(Autosomal dominant susceptibility
to fungal nail infection)

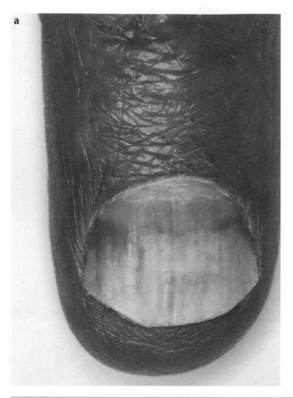
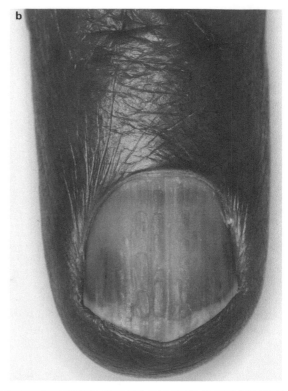

■ FIGURE 8.7

(a) Psoriatic onycholysis limited to the nails and associated with *Trichophyton rubrum*. (b) The same patient after intermittent treatment with itraconazole (two pulses).

■■■ REFERENCES

1. Götz H, Patiri C, Hantschke D. Das Wachstum von Dermatophyten auf normalem und psoriatischem Nagelkeratin. Mykosen 1974; 17: 373–7.
2. Feuerman E, Alteras I, Aryelly J. The incidence of pathogenic fungi in psoriatic nails. Castellania 1976; 4: 195–6.
3. Staberg B, Gammeltoft MD, Onsberg P. Onychomycosis in patients with psoriasis. Acta Derma Venereol 1983; 63: 436–8.
4. Fransson J, Stogards K, Hammar H. Palmoplantar lesions in psoriatic patients and their relation to inverse psoriasis, tinea infection and contact allergy. Acta Derma Venereol 1985; 65: 218–22.
5. Malka N, Contet-Audonnet N, Reichert-Penetrat S, Truchetet F, Barbaud A, Schmutz JL. Onychomycoses et psoriasis unguéal. J Mycol Méd 1998; 8: 192–5.
6. Ständer H, Ständer M, Nolting S. Häufigkeit des Pilzbefalles bei Nagelpsoriasis. Hautarzt 2001; 52: 418–22.
7. Gupta AK, Lynde CW, Jain HC, et al. A higher prevalence of onychomycosis in psoriatics compared with non-psoriatics: a multicentre study. Br J Dermatol 1997; 136: 786–9.
8. Kjellberg-Rarsen G, Haederstal M, Svejgaard EL. The prevalence of onychomycosis in patients with psoriasis and other skin diseases. Acta Derma Venereol 2003; 83: 206–9.
9. Haneke E: Nail biopsies in onychomycosis. Mykosen 1985; 28: 473–80.
10. Haneke E: Bedeutung der Nagelhistologie für die Diagnostik und Therapie der Onychomykosen. Ärztl Kosmetol 1988; 18: 248–54.
11. Haneke E. Pathogenesis of onychomycoses. Dermatology 1998; 197: 200–1.
12. Lawry M, Haneke E, Storbeck K, et al. Methods for diagnosing onychomycosis: A comparative study and review of the literature. Arch Dermatol 2000; 136: 1112–26.
13. Kemma ME, Elewski BE. A US epidemiologic survey of superficial fungal diseases. J Am Acad Dermatol 1996; 35;539–42.

14. Williams HC. The epidemiology of onychomycosis in Britain. Br J Dermatol 1993; 129: 101–9.

15. Baran RL. A nail psoriasis severity index. Br J Dermatol. 2004; 150: 568–9.

16. Feuilhade de Chauvin M, Lacroix C. Differential diagnosis of onychomycosis. Ann Dermatol Venereol 2003; 130: 1248–53 [in French].

17. Fletcher CL, Hay RJ, Smeeton NC. Observer agreement in recording the clinical signs of nail disease and the accuracy of a clinical diagnosis of fungal and non-fungal nail disease. Br J Dermatol 2003; 148: 558–62.

Chapter 9

The painful nail

Pain is a common nonspecific symptom of many conditions of and around the nail. It may indicate inflammation, trauma, or a tumor. It is often the reason to consult a physician. Despite its lack of specificity, the quality of the pain may sometimes give a hint as to the correct diagnosis. Precise localization of the pain, either spontaneous or upon palpation or probing, may further aid in reaching a diagnosis.

The nail plate covers a virtual space, which is strictly limited inwardly by the bone and periosteum, by the nail folds and the onychocorneal band to the sides, and above. The nail plate is very firmly attached to the nail bed, and less firmly to the matrix. Similar conditions are found between the dermis of the nail bed and matrix and the underlying periosteum and bone of the terminal phalanx. The nail apparatus is also very richly innervated, receiving approximately 60% of the digital nerves. Interestingly, however, the pressure pain threshold has been found to be higher over the nail bed than over bony prominences and muscles; it is higher on the feet than on the hands.[1] In addition, the distal interphalangeal joint may be inflamed, infected, or otherwise painful.

The diagnosis of a painful nail requires an accurate patient history, including former diseases and medications, possible trauma, hobbies, and profession. Particular attention has to be paid to the pain characteristics:

- onset of the pain
- course
- intensity
- nature
- response to alterations of blood circulation, temperature, etc.
- response to treatment with particular drugs

■■■ PATIENT EXAMINATION

All parts of the nail mentioned above have to be examined and compared with the neighboring digits and the contralateral nail. Any modifications in size, color, shape, periungual tissues, tenderness, temperature, and circumference have to be precisely explored. This is done with the digit in a relaxed and forced extended position, as well as pressed on a hard surface to allow alterations in blood supply to be noted. A magnifying lens or surgical microscope aids in noting fine alterations. Palpation following inspection permits one to diagnose any modification in the consistency of periungual tissues, and may also intensify the pain when a certain region is palpated. This is then more accurately localized by using a blunt probe. Diascopy allows the true color of the digit to be seen as the glass spatula presses out the red color from the capillaries. Transillumination with a spotlight makes a lesion shine when it is cystic and filled with a clear fluid or form a shadow in the case of a foreign body. Dermatoscopy is of great help for the differential diagnosis of pigments, particularly to differentiate blood from melanin and microbial pigments. An X-ray is mandatory in the case of a severe trauma or when the pain from a supposedly minor trauma does not disappear in due course. Ultrasoft X-rays, particularly xeroradiography with magnification, also permit some soft tissue outlines to be seen in relation to the bone. Magnetic resonance tomography is a useful tool to localize glomus tumors and other vascular alterations as well as lesions rich in fluids. Biopsy with histopathological examination is the gold standard of all diagnostic measures.

Pain is a very subjective symptom, and varies from person to person. Some individuals are unconcerned, while others complain of unbearable pain. It is therefore wise to accurately examine the clinical signs and try to relate them to the intensity and nature of pain.

Pain should be classified as being due to:

- infection (Table 9.1)
- trauma (Table 9.2)
- inflammation (Table 9.3)
- foreign bodies (Table 9.4)
- tumors (Table 9.5)

However, there may be some overlap.

Psoriasis, although the most frequent dermatosis affecting the nail, has only rarely been examined as a cause of pain as it is usually thought not to be characteristically painful. De Jong et al[2] assessed ungual psoriasis associated with disability. Of 7000 questionnaires, 1728 were returned that were suitable for evaluation (25%). Joint complaints existed in 48.5% of patients. A remarkably high percentage of patients suffered from pain caused by psoriatic nail changes (51.8%). This percentage is comparable to what was found in quality-of-life investigations in onychomycosis.[3,4] The subungual hyperkeratosis that may be found in both the fingers and the toes may not only interfere with

■ TABLE 9.1

Infection as a cause of painful nails

Disease	Nature of pain
Onychomycosis	Pain due to massive subungual hyperkeratosis, particularly when tight shoes are worn.
	Painful perionyxis in nondermatophyte mold infection.[6,7] (Figure 9.1)
Acute paronychia	Moderate (Figure 9.2)
Bacterial nail bed infection	Moderate (Figure 9.3)
Chronic paronychia	Subacute flare painful
Felon	Often pulsating, decreases when extremity is raised (Figure 9.4)
Osteitis terminalis	Chronic intense pain
Bulla repens (runaround)	Staphylococcal infection, mild pain
Deep pyogenic infection	Often pulsating
Erysipeloid	Chronic mild to moderate pain
Herpes simplex (herpetic whitlow)	Intense pain, often before visible vesicles, commonly preceding lymphangitis. Often recurring (Figures 9.5 and 9.6)
Ulcerative leishmaniasis	Chronic pain from ulcer[8]

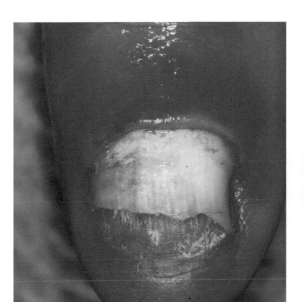

■ FIGURE 9.1

Tender paronychia associated with proximal leukonychia due to *Aspergillus* spp.

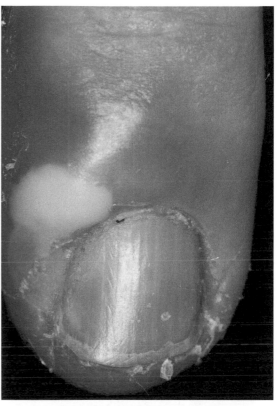

■ FIGURE 9.2

Acute paronychia with a bulla of pus.

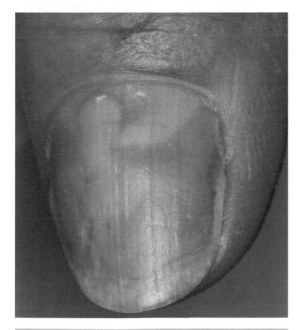

■ FIGURE 9.3

Bacterial nail bed infection.

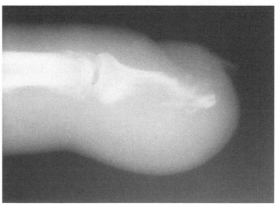

■ FIGURE 9.4

Felon X-rays. (Courtesy of WA Murphy and B Monsees, USA.)

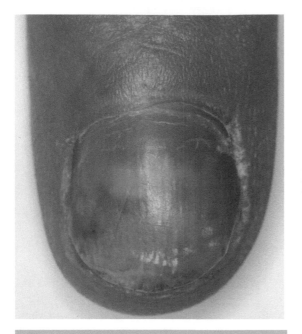

■ **FIGURE 9.5**

Recurrent subungual herpes.

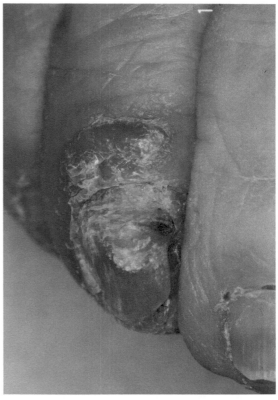

■ **FIGURE 9.7**

Psoriatic arthropathy.

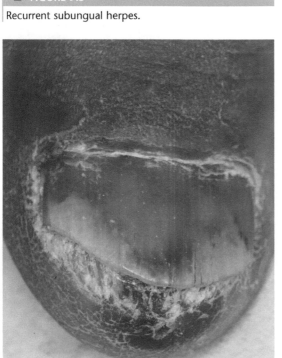

■ **FIGURE 9.6**

Herpes associated with psoriatic finger.

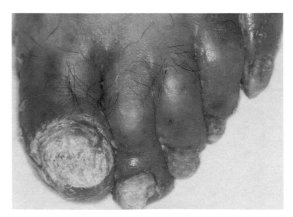

■ **FIGURE 9.8**

Psoriatic onychopachydermoperiostitis.

■ **TABLE 9.2**

Trauma-induced nail pain

Condition	Nature of pain
Ungual psoriasis	About one-half of patients have pain[2,3]
Psoriatic athropathy, including	Weather-dependent, usually mild to moderate[9,10]
psoriatic onychopachydermoperiostitis	Occasionally severe pain[11,12] (Figures 9.7 and 9.8)
Reiter syndrome	Moderate chronic pain (Figure 9.9)
Allergic contact dermatitis to	Painful pruritic vesicles on perionychium[13]
artificial nails	
Dorsolateral fissure of the	Painful fissure, particularly in winter and dry conditions[14]
fingertip	(Figure 9.10)
Lichenoid graft-versus-host	Dystrophic nails may become painful[15]
disease	
Ulcerative lichen planus	Slowly developing pain, depending on severity of ulceration and
	nail dystrophy[16] (Figure 9.11)
Systemic lupus erythematosus	Painful red lunulae[17]
Sarcoidosis (osteitis)	Variable
Thromboangiitis obliterans of	Painful ulceration[18,19]
the digital arteries	
Acro-osteolysis	Often surprisingly painless, despite tremendous destruction of distal
	phalanx and nail organ, because of sensory neuropathy
Nail side-effect of taxanes	Moderate to intense pain, subungual hemorrhagic abscess
	formation, brownish nail discoloration, pus-like discharge from
	under the nail[20–22]
Periungual inflammation due	Painful paronychia[23,24] often with granulation tissue
to retinoids, antiretrovirals,	
epidermal growth factor inhibitors	
Repeated microtrauma	Development of painful bullae under the nail[25] in photo-onycholysis
Ingrown nail	See Table 9.4
Periungual telangiectasias	Painful telangiectasias[26]
in AIDS	
Acute radiodermatitis	Chronic (Figure 9.12)
Pachydermoperiostosis	Moderate pain[27]
Subclavian occlusion	Painful nail[28]

■ **TABLE 9.3**

Painful nail due to noninfectious inflammation

Condition	Nature of pain
Crush injury, hammer blow	Acute intense pain, pulsating at the beginning. Subungual hematoma, small area of leukoplakia over the site of injury visible after 2 weeks[29,30]
Splinter	Variable, often more intense with pain due to late infection (Figure 9.13)
Repeated shearing trauma	Dull pain, prehyponychial hematoma
Ski-boot, tennis, surfer's toe	Variable. Often nonmigratory hematoma under lateral portion of hallux nail
Cold injury	Pain during rewarming
Hydrofluoric acid burn	Severe pain and deep tissue destruction[31] (Figure 9.14)
Onychomadesis after splint removal	Painful swelling of proximal nail folds with erythema[32]
Subungual heloma (corn)	Due to chronic pressure and friction, pain on pressure, tight shoe wear (Figure 9.15)
Onychophosis	Due to chronic pressure in lateral nail groove, tight shoes cause pain (Figure 9.16)
Pincer nail	Very variable: from none to excruciating (Figure 9.17)
Postoperative pain	Depending on extent and type of surgery, pain developing later than 24–48 hours after surgery may indicate postoperative infection. Change of dressing[33]
Complex regional pain syndrome/sympathic reflex dystrophy	Slowly increasing discomfort and pain, usually after digital or nail surgery[34]
Brittle nails	Sometimes painful[35]
Photo-onycholysis	Often painful[36] (without any trauma)
Photo-hemorrhages	Painful (Figure 9.18)
Pterygium inversum	Painful on mechanical strain, sometimes also spontaneously[37] (Figure 9.19)
Pachyonychia congenita tarda	Pain of toenails[38]

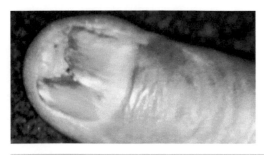

■ **FIGURE 9.9**

Reiter syndrome.

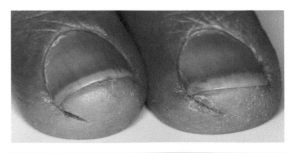

■ **FIGURE 9.10**

Dorsolateral fissure of the fingertip.

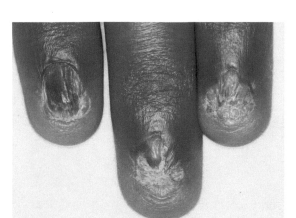

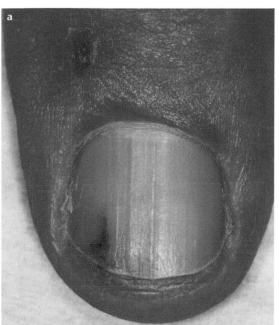

■ FIGURE 9.11

Ulcerative lichen planus.

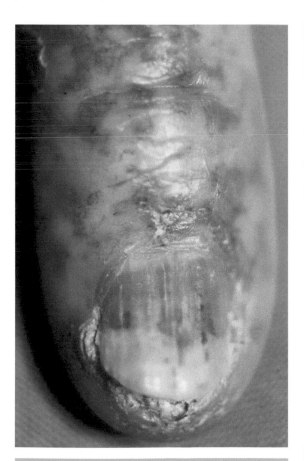

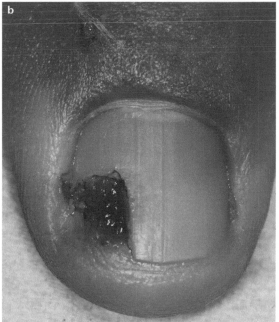

■ FIGURE 9.12

Acute radiodermatitis on a psoriatic digit.

■ FIGURE 9.13

(a) Splinter of the distal nail bed. (b) The same patient after removal of splinter.

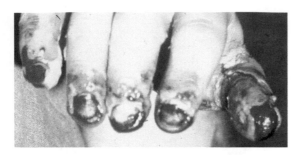

■ FIGURE 9.14

Hydrofluoric acid burn of the digit. (Courtesy of G Sebastian, Germany.)

manual dexterity, but also cause pain upon pressure and certain movements, and in the feet also during gait or with wearing of tight shoes.[5] Psoriatic arthritis is also usually painful, as is the distal phalanx in Reiter syndrome.

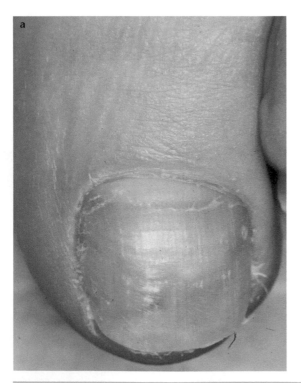
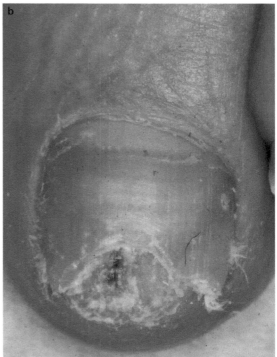

■ FIGURE 9.15

Heloma before partial nail avulsion. Exposure of the distal nail bed.

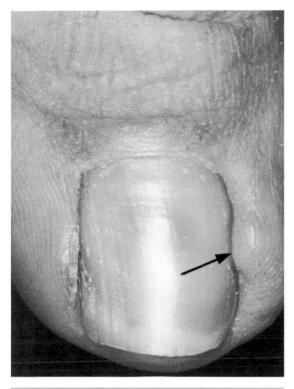

Onychophosis of the lateral nail fold.

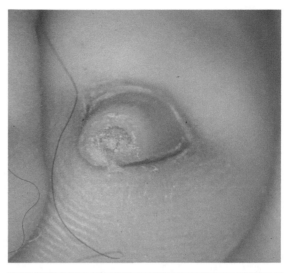

■ FIGURE 9.17
Pincer nail.

■ TABLE 9.4	
Foreign bodies	
Condition	**Nature of pain**
Splinter	Variable (see Table 9.3 and Figure 9.13)[39]
Ingrown nail	Nail plate spicule pierces skin of nail groove and induces pain, which is intensified by secondary infection. Many tumors and metastases may mimic an ingrown nail[40,41]
Congenital hypertrophy of the lateral nail fold	Pain due to ingrowing nail[42]
Ectopic nail	Ectopic nail may be very painful during gait when located on the sole of the foot[43]

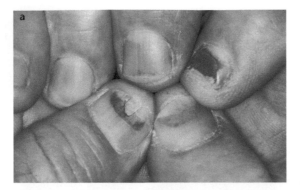

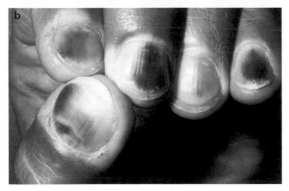

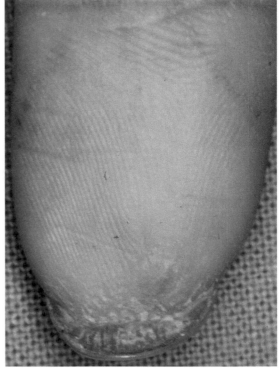

■ **FIGURE 9.18**

(a) Photo-onycholysis type I involving almost all of the fingers. (b) Photo-hemorrhages following PUVA therapy.

■ **FIGURE 9.19**

Pterygium inversum associated with acrosclerosis.

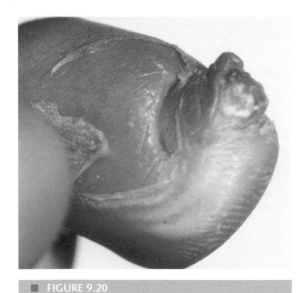

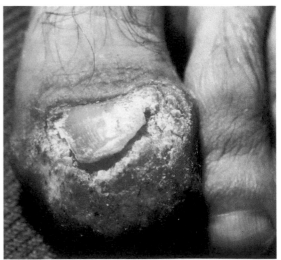

■ **FIGURE 9.20**

Subungual exostosis lifting up the distal nail plate.

■ **FIGURE 9.21**

Tender subungual and periungual wart.

■ **TABLE 9.5**

Tumor-induced pain of the nail apparatus

Condition	Nature of pain
Glomus tumor	Throbbing intense pain radiating up to the shoulder intensifies upon pressure, shock and cold; disappears when tourniquet with pressure over systolic blood pressure is applied[14,16, 44–46]
	Reappearance of pain after surgery indicates a recurrence[47]
Arteriovenous malformation	Painful hyperkeratotic nodule with fissures; pain subsides after sclerotherapy[48]
Keratoacanthoma	Rapidly growing tumor with slowly increasing pain intensity due to bone erosion and space-occupying growth[49–52]
Subungual tumors of incontinentia pigmenti	Longstanding, painful lesions[53–59]
Osteoid osteoma	Nagging pain, irregular nightly pain attacks, good response to acetylsalicylic acid (aspirin) and naproxen[60]
Exostosis, osteochondroma	Mainly pain on touch, pressure, during sports activities[61–63] (Figure 9.20)
Enchondroma	Dull pain, more intense pain due to pathological fracture[64]
Myxoid pseudocyst	Sometimes painful;[65] pain due to degenerative osteoarthritis of the distal interphalangeal joint[66]
Aneurysmal bone cyst	Painful intraosseous arteriovenous fistula with rapid growth, bulbous enlargement of the fingertip of young persons[67]
Epidermoid cyst	May be painful upon pressure, rarely spontaneously[68]
Fibroma, fibrokeratomas, Koenen's tumors	Rarely painful[69]
Leiomyoma	Painful on pressure and cold
Metastases of internal carcinomas	Pain due to osteolytic process, swelling or ingrown nail[40,70]
Squamous cell carcinoma	Late symptom
Neurofibroma	Usually asymptomatic
Post-traumatic neuroma	Spontaneous pain or on pressure, touch
Subungual wart	Pain due to space-occupying growth (Figure 9.21)
Cirsoid angioma	Moderate pain
Giant cell tumor of the bone	Pain that is suddenly noted in hand, tender to palpation[71,72]
Melanoma	May mimic ingrown nail
Clear cell syringofibroadenoma	Intermittent pain[73]
Chondrosarcoma	Pain and swelling common[74]
Phalangeal sarcoma	Extremely painful due to enlargement of the distal phalanx[75]
Epithelioid sarcoma	Occasionally pain and tenderness[76]
Epithelioid leimyosarcoma	Diffuse pain[77]

■■■ REFERENCES

1. Rölke R, Andrews Campbell K, Magerl W, Treede RD. Deep pain thresholds in the distal limbs of healthy human subjects. Eur J Pain 2005; 9: 39–48.
2. De Jong EM, Seegers BA, Gulinck MK, Boezeman JB, Van de Kerkhof PC. Psoriasis of the nails associated with disability in a large number of patients: results of a recent interview with 1,728 patients. Dermatology 1996; 193: 300–3.
3. Lubeck DP, Gause D, Schein JR, Prebil LE, Potter LP. A health-related quality of life measure for use in patients with onychomycosis: a validation study. Qual Life Res 1999; 8: 121–9.
4. Drake LA, Patrick DL, Fleckman P, et al. The impact of onychomycosis on quality of life: development of an international onychomycosis-specific questionnaire to measure patient quality of life. J Am Acad Dermatol 1999; 41: 189–96.
5. Sanchez Regana M, Martin Ezquerra G, Umbert Millet P, Llambi Mateos F. Treatment of nail psoriasis with 8% clobetasol nail lacquer: positive experience in 10 patients. J Eur Acad Dermatol Venereol 2005; 19: 573–7.
6. Tosti A, Piraccini BM, Stinchi C, Lorenzi S. Onychomycosis due to *Scopulariopsis brevicaulis*: clinical features and response to systemic antifungals. Br J Dermatol 1996; 135: 799–802.
7. Gianni C, Romano C. Clinical and histological aspects of toenail onychomycosis caused by *Aspergillus* spp.: 34 cases treated with weekly intermittent terbinafine. Dermatology 2004; 209: 104–10.
8. Ogawa MM, Macedo FS, Alchorne MM, Tomimori-Yamashita J. Unusual location of cutaneous leishmaniasis on the hallux in a Brazilian patient. Int J Dermatol 2002; 41: 439–40.
9. Schröder K, Goerdt S, Sieper J, et al. Psoriatic onycho-pachydermo-periostitis (POPP). Hautarzt 1997; 48: 500–3
10. Kroiss MM, Vogt T, Finkenzeller T, Landthaler M, Stolz W. Psoriatic onycho-pachydermo-periostitis. Z Rheumatol 2002; 61: 598–600.
11. Ziemer A, Heider M, Göring HD. Psoriasiform onychopachydermoperiostitis of the large toes: the OP3GO syndrome. Hautarzt 1998; 49: 859–62.
12. Jury CS, Fleming C, Kemmett D. Severe nail dystrophy associated with painful fingertips. Diagnosis: psoriatic onychopachydermoperiostitis (POPP). Arch Dermatol 2000; 136: 925–30.
13. Mowad CM, Ferringer T. Allergic contact dermatitis from acrylates in artificial nails. Dermatitis 2004; 15: 51–3.
14. Dawber R, Baran R. Painful dorso-lateral fissure of the fingertip – an extension of the lateral nail groove. Clin Exp Dermatol 1984; 9: 419–20.
15. Palencia SI, Rodriguez-Peralto JL, Castano E, Vanaclocha F, Iglesias L. Lichenoid nail changes as sole external manifestation of graft vs. host disease. Int J Dermatol 2002;.41: 44–5.
16. Isogai Z, Koashi Y, Sunohara A, Tsuji T. Ulcerative lichen planus: a rare variant of lichen planus. J Dermatol 1997; 24: 270–2.
17. Garcia-Patos V, Bartralot R, Ordi J, et al. Systemic lupus erythematosus presenting with red lunulae. J Am Acad Dermatol 1997; 36: 834–6.
18. Quenneville JG, Gossard D. Subungueal–splinter hemorrhage: an early sign of thromboangiitis obliterans. Angiology 1981; 32: 424–32.
19. Brosky ME, Zaki HS, Studer SP. The use of protective digit prostheses in management of microangiopathy of fingers. J Prosthet Dent 1999; 82: 246–8.
20. Wasner G, Hilpert F, Schattschneider J, et al. Docetaxel-induced nail changes – a neurogenic mechanism: a case report. J Neurooncol 2002; 58: 167–74.
21. Nicolopoulos J, Howard A. Docetaxel-induced nail dystrophy. Australas J Dermatol 2002; 43: 293–6.
22. Ghetti E, Piraccini BM, Tosti A. Onycholysis and subungual haemorrhages secondary to systemic chemotherapy (paclitaxel). J Eur Acad Dermatol Venereol 2003; 17: 459–60.
23. Tosti A, Piraccini BM, D'Antuono A, Marzaduri S, Bettoli V. Paronychia associated with antiretroviral therapy. Br J Dermatol 1999; 140: 1165–8.
24. Baran R. Pyogenic granuloma-like lesions associated with topical retinoid therapy. J Am Acad Dermatol 2002; 47: 970.
25. Ibsen HH, Lasthein Andersen B. Photo-onycholysis due to tetracycline-hydrochloride. Acta Derma Venereol 1983; 63: 555–7.
26. Ruiz-Avila P, Tercedor J, Fuentes E, Villar A, Rodenas JM. Painful periungual telangiectasias in a patient with acquired immunodeficiency syndrome. Int J Dermatol 1995; 34: 199–200.
27. Bhaskaranand K, Shetty RR, Bhat AK. Pachydermoperiostosis: three case reports. J Orthop Surg (Hong Kong) 2001; 9: 61–6.
28. Kerdel FA, Baden HP. Subclavian occlusive disease presenting as a painful nail. J Am Acad Dermatol 1984; 10: 523–5.
29. Brown RE. Acute nail bed injuries. Hand Clin 2002; 18: 561–75.
30. Wang QC, Johnson BA. Fingertip injuries. Am Fam Physician 2001; 63: 1961–6.
31. Vance MV, Curry SC, Kunkel DB, Ryan PJ, Ruggeri SB. Digital hydrofluoric acid burns: treatment with intraarterial calcium infusion. Ann Emerg Med 1986; 15: 890–6.
32. Kim HS, Lee SH, Yoon TJ, Oh CW, Kim TH. Early stage onychomadesis presenting as painful swellings of proximal nail folds. Cutis 2001; 67: 317–18.
33. King B. Pain at first dressing change after toenail avulsion: the experience of nurses, patients and an observer: 1. J Wound Care 2003; 12: 5–10.
34. Linchitz RM, Raheb JC. Subcutaneous infusion of lidocaine provides effective pain relief for CRPS patients. Clin J Pain 1999; 15: 67–72.
35. van de Kerkhof PC, Pasch MC, Scher RK, et al. Brittle nail syndrome: a pathogenesis-based approach with a proposed grading system. J Am Acad Dermatol 2005; 53: 644–51.
36. Baran R, Juhlin L. Photoonycholysis. Photoderm Photoimmunol Photomed 2002; 18: 202–7.
37. Christophers E. Familiäre subunguale Pterygien. Hautarzt 1975; 26: 543–4.

38. Hannaford RS, Stapleton K. Pachyonychia congenita tarda. Australas J Dermatol 2000; 41: 175–7.
39. Chan C, Salam GA. Splinter removal. Am Fam Physician 2003; 67: 2557–62.
40. Amiot RA, Wilson SE, Reznicek MJ, Webb BS. Endometrial carcinoma metastasis to the distal phalanx of the hallux: a case report. J Foot Ankle Surg 2005; 44: 462–5.
41. Farley-Sakevich T, Grady JF, Zager E, Axe TM. Onychoplasty with carbon dioxide laser matrixectomy for treatment of ingrown toenails. J Am Podiatr Med Assoc 2005; 95: 175–9.
42. Piraccini BM, Parente GL, Varotti E, Tosti A. Congenital hypertrophy of the lateral nail folds of the hallux: clinical features and follow-up of seven cases. Pediatr Dermatol 2000; 17: 348–51.
43. Ena P, Mazzarello V, Dessy LA. Relapsing and painful horny excrescence of the sole: a case of ectopic plantar nail. Eur J Dermatol 2004; 14: 51.
44. Sheils WC, Becton JL, Christian JD. Subungual glomus tumor: a cause of pain beneath the finger nail. J Med Ass Georgia 1972; 64: 268–70.
45. De Maerteleire W, Naetens P, De Smet L. Glomus tumors. Acta Orthop Belg 2000; 66: 169–73.
46. Özdemir O, Coskunol E, Özalp T, Özaksar K. Glomus tumors of the finger: a report on 60 cases. Acta Orthop Traumatol Turc 2003; 37: 244–8.
47. Takata H, Ikuta Y, Ishida O, Kimori K. Treatment of subungual glomus tumour. Hand Surg 2001; 6: 25–7.
48. Park CO, Lee MJ, Chung KY. Treatment fo unusual vascular lesions: usefulness of sclerotherapy in lymphangioma circumscriptum and acquired digital arteriovenous malformation. Dermatol Surg 2005; 31: 1451–3.
49. Levy DW, Bonakdarpour A, Putong PB, Mesgarzadeh M, Betz RR. Subungual keratoacanthoma. Skeletal Radiol 1985; 13: 287–90.
50. Bräuninger W, Hoede N. Subunguales Keratoakanthom. Hautarzt 1986; 37: 270–3.
51. Wiemers S, Stengel R, Schöpf E, Laaff H. Subunguales Keratoakanthom. Hautarzt 1994; 45: 25–8.
52. Oliwiecki S, Peachey RD, Bradfield JW, Ellis J, Lovell CR. Subungual keratoacanthoma – a report of four cases and review of the literature. Clin Exp Dermatol 1994; 19: 230–5.
53. Aguadé JP, Mascaró JM, Herrero C, Castel T. Painful and spontaneously healing subungual dyskeratotic tumors; their relation to incontinentia pigmenti. Ann Dermatol Syphiligr (Paris) 1973; 100: 159–68.
54. Mascaró JM, Palou J, Vives P. Painful subungual keratotic tumors in incontinentia pigmenti. J Am Acad Dermatol 1985; 13: 913–18.
55. Simmons DA, Kegel MF, Scher RK, Hines YC. Subungual tumors in incontinentia pigmenti. Arch Dermatol 1986; 122: 1431–4.
56. Adeniran A, Townsend PL, Peachey RD. Incontinentia pigmenti (Bloch–Sulzberger syndrome) manifesting as painful periungual and subungual tumours. J Hand Surg 1993; 18: 667–9.
57. Abimelec P, Rybojad M, Cambiaghi S, et al. Late, painful, subungual hyperkeratosis in incontinentia pigmenti. Pediatr Dermatol 1995; 12: 340–2.
58. Malvehy J, Palou J, Mascaro JM. Painful subungual tumour in incontinentia pigmenti. Response to treatment with etretinate. Br J Dermatol 1998; 138: 554–5.
59. Montes CM, Maize JC, Guerry-Force ML. Incontinentia pigmenti with painful subungual tumors: a two-generation study. J Am Acad Dermatol 2004; 50(Suppl): S45–52.
60. Saville PD. A medical option for the treatment of osteoid osteoma. Arthr Rheumat 1980; 23: 1409–11.
61. Rutkai K, Daroczy J. Subunguale Exostose. Hautarzt 1986; 37: 402–4.
62. Jetmalani SN, Rich P, White CR Jr. Painful solitary subungual nodule. Subungual exostosis (SE). Arch Dermatol 1992; 128: 849–52.
63. Tüzüner T, Kavak A, Ustundag N, Parlak AH. A painful subungual nodule: subungual exostosis. Acta Orthop Traumatol Turc 2004; 38: 71–4.
64. Shimizu K, Kotoura Y, Nishijima N, Nakamura T. Enchondroma of the distal phalanx of the hand. J Bone Joint Surg Am 1997; 79: 898–900.
65. Lonsdale-Eccles AA, Langtry JA. Treatment of digital myxoid cysts with infrared coagulation: a retrospective case series. Br J Dermatol 2005; 153: 972–5.
66. Derks DH, Koch AR. Favorable results of surgical treatment of mucoid cysts of the fingers and thumb in 20 patients, Leyenburg Hospital, Den Haag, 1992–99. Ned Tijdschr Geneeskd 2000; 144: 1314–18.
67. Schajowicz F, Aiello F, Slulittel I. Cystic and pseudocystic lesions of the terminal phalanx with special reference to epidermoid cysts. Clin Orthop Rel Res 1970; 68: 84–92.
68. Yung CW, Estes SA. Subungual epidermal cyst. J Am Acad Dermatol 1980; 3: 599–601.
69. Griffith T, Lezama JL, Sanders S, Adelman HM. A man with a history of skin lesions and seizures. Hosp Pract (Off Ed) 2001; 36: 15–16.
70. Cohen PR. Metastatic tumors to the nail unit: subungual metastases. Dermatol Surg 2001; 27: 280–93.
71. Averill RM, Smith RJ, Campbell CJ. Giant-cell tumors of the bones of the hand. J Hand Surg 1980; 5: 39–50.
72. Goettmann S, Baran R, Fraitag S. Tumeurs à cellules géantes osseuses avec atteinte unguéale. Ann Dermatol Venereol 1995; 122 (Suppl 1): S148–9.
73. Fouilloux B, Perrin C, Dutoit M, Cambazard F. Clear cell syringofibroadenoma (of Mascaro) of the nail. Br J Dermatol 2001; 144: 625–7.
74. Gargan TJ, Kanter W, Wolfort FG. Multiple chondrosarcomas of the hand. Ann Plast Surg 1984; 12: 542–6.
75. Marcove RC, Charosky CB. Phalangeal sarcomas simulating infections of the digits. Clin Orthop Rel Res 1972; 83: 224–31.
76. Tsoitis G, Asvesti Z, Papadimitriou C. Epithelioid sarcoma. In: Book of Abstracts, European Society of Pediatric Dermatology, Rotterdam: 1996, 133 (Abst 86).
77. Bryant J. Subungual epithelioid leiomyosarcoma. South Med J 1992; 85: 560–1.

Chapter 10

Tumors and swellings: lumps and bumps in the nail area

Swellings due to tumors, inflammation, infection, or deposition of certain materials are frequent. However, they occur relatively rarely in psoriasis or onychomycosis, and when observed they are usually diffuse and not circumscribed tumors.

Chronic paronychia in psoriasis and onychomycosis and distal interphalangeal psoriatic arthritis are the most common causes (see Chapter 5). However, paronychia-like swellings may also occur in Reiter syndrome and a variety of tumors.

Psoriatic onychopachydermoperiostitis (Figure 10.1) is characterized by psoriatic nail changes, thickening of the distal soft tissues with osteoperiostitis of the terminal phalanx, but without alterations of the distal interphalangeal joint. This condition mainly involves the big toe,[1] rarely the fingers.[2] Pain, varying from moderate to severe, is a consistent feature. Although joint changes are characteristically lacking, this particular form of psoriasis is considered a variant of psoriatic arthritis.[3]

As there are many different conditions that may cause tumors and/or swellings of the distal phalanx, we have tried to classify them here according to certain clinical signs and symptoms as well as to their localization at the tip of the digit. It is important to note that pain is an entirely subjective symptom. Therefore, some lesions will be listed more than once, under different headings.

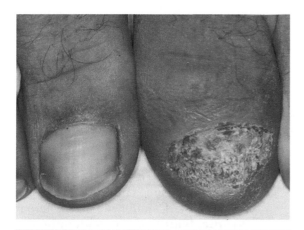

Psoriatic onychopachydermoperiostitis.

■■■ SWELLINGS WITHOUT SIGNS OF INFLAMMATION
(Table 10.1)

A rudimentary **hexadactyly** may be localized at the distal phalanx, usually of the little finger, and may look like a small tumor as well as an **ectopic nail**[4] (Figure 10.2) The subungual hyperkeratosis in pachyonychia congenita may also be mistaken for a subungual tumor.

Many **neoplasms** come without an inflammatory erythema. They may be localized under the nail or in the periungual soft tissue and may be firm, elastic, or soft. Depending on the

Swelling and tumors without signs of inflammation

Diagnosis	Signs	Symptoms
Viral warts	Round to oval, hard nodules with a rough, keratotic surface; may fissure and become secondarily inflamed	Pain when localized under nail or when fissured.
Subungual exostosis	Stone-hard nodule that lifts the nail up when located under the hyponychium	Often pain
Myxoid pseudocyst	Usually in proximal nail fold, sometimes next to the distal interphalangeal joint, round, dome-shaped, skin-colored to glassy, cystic lesion, elastic or flaccid; tends to penetrate into cul-de-sac through rupture of undersurface of proximal nail folds; causes longitudinal depression that may be very irregular in the case of rupture. In subungual location, hemiovercurvature of the nail and characteristic violaceous transparent lesion	Usually asymptomatic. If pain, then usually due to to degenerative osteoarthritis of the distal interphalangeal joint with Heberden nodes.
Synovioma	Irregular hard tumor when located on the dorsal aspect of the distal phalanx. Diffuse swelling of the tip when located in the palmar aspect, sometimes with pseudoclubbing	Usually none

localization, they may characteristically change their shape, as is for instance seen in common **warts** (Figure 10.3), which present as round protuberant nodules on the proximal nail fold and are usually at the level of the surrounding skin on the tip of the digit and pulp, but more oval on the lateral nail folds. They may lift up the nail plate when they occur in the distal nail bed. Along the hyponychium, they may present as a linear hyperkeratosis, which becomes obvious only after immersion in water, following hydration of the hyperkeratosis that covers the wart. Occasionally, they may exhibit very large dimensions and distort the nail growth.

Erythema and swelling have been described in **Langerhans cell histiocytosis** of the Letterer–Siwe and Hand–Schüller–Christian types of histiocytosis X. They may resemble chronic paronychia (Figure 10.4), although they are usually accompanied by subungual hyperkeratosis, onycholysis, and/or subungual purpura.[5]

Chronic lymphocytic leukemia (Figure 10.5) may produce specific infiltrates of the proximal and lateral nail folds resembling

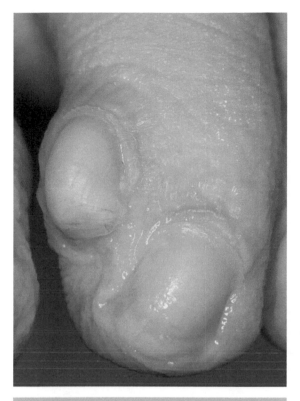

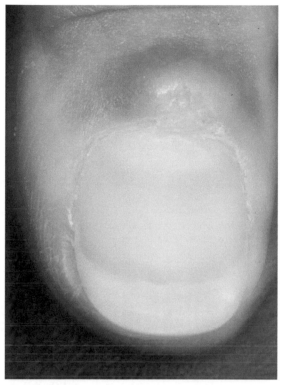

■ FIGURE 10.2

Rudimentary hexadactyly.

■ FIGURE 10.3

Protuberant nodule on the proximal nail fold: warts.

paronychia,[6] and subungual infiltrates have even been seen.

Myelomonocytic leukemia can produce an infiltration of the distal phalanx of the thumb, resulting in a chronic whitlow with bone involvement.

We have seen a brownish infiltrate in the proximal nail fold of a patient suffering from **chronic myelocytic leukemia**. However, considering the frequency of leukemias as a whole, nail involvement is rare.

An asymptomatic subungual nodule has been seen in a patient with **plasmacytoma.**[7]

Although **mycosis fungoides** (Figure 10.6) when affecting the nail commonly induces non-specific nail dystrophy, it rarely causes a nodular infiltrate. A case of an elephantiasis-like enlargement of the middle finger and multiple nodular

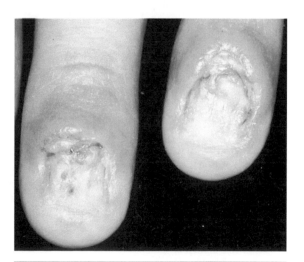

■ FIGURE 10.4

Paronychia in Langerhans cell histiocytosis. (Courtesy of T Bieber, Germany.)

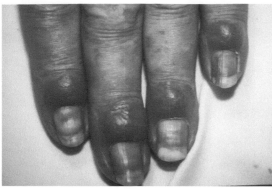

Chronic lymphocytic leukemia. (Courtesy of HA Luscombe, USA).

lesions on the fingers has been observed in a 56-year-old patient.[8]

Tophi of **gout** (Figure 10.7) can produce circumscribed tumors around the nail and lead to distortion of the nail apparatus and even psoriasiform nail changes.

Extensive tuberous **xanthomas** on the finger have been observed in type III hyperlipoproteinemia and **tendon xanthomas of the extensor tendons** (Figure 10.8) of the fingers in cerebrotendinous xanthomatosis. Familial hypercholesterolemic xanthomatosis have caused pseudo-Koenen tumors in the toes of a patient.

A subungual **xanthogranuloma** (Figure 10.9) elevating the index fingernail plate of a 30-month-old boy with partial destruction of the nail plate has also been observed.[9]

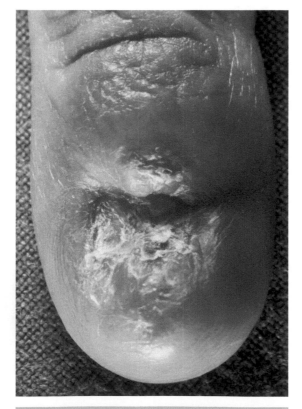

■ FIGURE 10.6

Mycoisis fungoides. (Courtesy of S Goettmann-Bonvallot, France.)

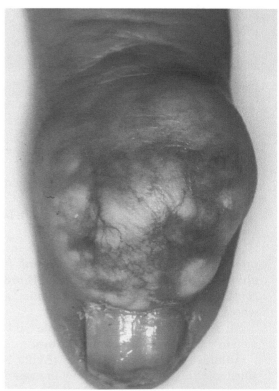

■ FIGURE 10.7

Tophus of gout. (Courtesy of G Canatta, Italy.)

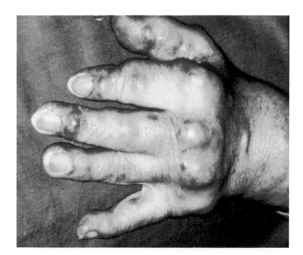

■ **FIGURE 10.8**

Extensor tendon xanthomas.

In **acro-osteopathia ulceromutilans**, the entire digit or the distal phalanx may be grossly enlarged, often in the big toenail (Figure 10.10). Most cases are acquired types due to alcoholic or diabetic peripheral neuropathy (Bureau–Barrière syndrome) although a number of hereditary neuropathy syndromes (e.g. Thévenard syndrome) also exist.

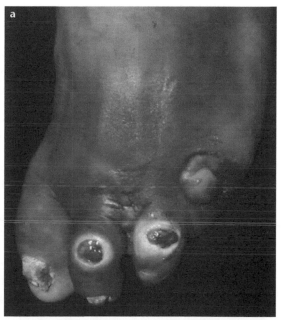

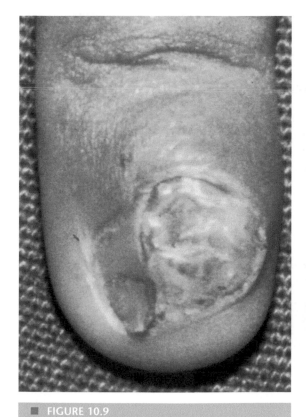

■ **FIGURE 10.9**

Subungual xanthogranuloma. (Courtesy of P Chang, Guatemala.)

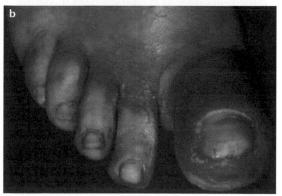

■ **FIGURE 10.10a,b**

Acropathia ulceromutilans. (Courtesy of B Dreno, France.)

Autosomal dominant **pachydermoperiostosis** (Figure 10.11) (primary or idiopathic pachydermoperiostosis, Uehlinger syndrome, Touraine–Solente–Golé syndrome) is characterized by pachydermia of the face, lower arms, and lower legs, and by hyperostosis of the tubular bones and along the ligaments of the small joints, including the distal interphalangeal joints, causing swelling and clubbing of nails as well as moderate pain unresponsive to treatment. Pachydermoperiostosis has also been seen as an associated feature in the Coffin–Siris, LEOPARD, and nail–patella syndromes.

Secondary pachydermoperiostosis (Marie–Bamberger syndrome) is a metabolically induced hyperostosis with digital clubbing seen in a variety of systemic diseases, the best known of which is the exophthalmos–myxoedema circumscriptum praetibiale–osteoarthropathia hypertrophicans syndrome (EMO complex).[10] Acromegaly may also cause swelling of the distal phalanx with pachydermoperiostosis-like features.

Hypertrophic pulmonary osteoarthropathy is linked to intrathoracic malignancies, either primary or metastatic. Lung cancer or metastases account for about 80% of cases, pleural neoplasms for 10%, and other intrathoracic tumors, brochiectases, empyema, lung abscesses, and other chronic lung infections for the remainder. It is characterized by digital clubbing, joint swellings, and new periosteal bone formation.

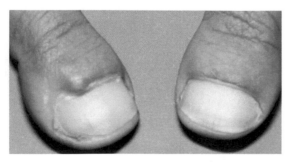

■ **FIGURE 10.11**

Pachydermoperiostosis. (Courtesy of PY Venencie, France.)

Pseudoclubbing may be observed in chronic mucocutaneous candiosis (Figure 10.12).

■■■ SWELLINGS WITH INFLAMMATION (EXCLUDING PARONYCHIA)

Inflammation may be clinically visible as erythema or may just be a histopathological phenomenon. It may be infectious or noninfectious.

In immunocompromised patients, particularly in AIDS, both **herpes simplex** (Figure 10.13) and **herpes zoster** (Figure 10.14) may occur as a verrucous generalized disease with circumscribed nodules also on the proximal nail fold.[11]

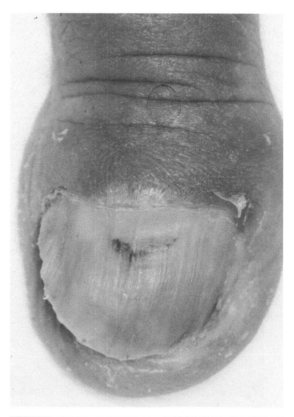

■ **FIGURE 10.12**

Pseudoclubbing in a treated CMCC patient.

Orf (ecthyma contagiosum) (Figure 10.15) and **milker's nodule** (Figure 10.16) are clinically similar infections caused by indistinguishable paravaccinia viruses. Orf is usually seen on the middle phalanx of the index finger, rarely on the distal phalanx adjacent to the nail, of persons working with sheep, goats, and reindeer, whereas milker's nodule is seen in farmers and veterinarians.[12] They present as tense blisters on an inflammatory nodule that slowly enlarges and usually tends to involute spontaneously.

A tumor-like granulomatous bacterial inflammation of the nail bed, **lectitis granulomatosa**, resembles bleeding subungual tumors and causes loss of the nail plate[13] (Figure 10.17).

Erysipeloid (Figure 10.18) due to *Erysipelothrix rhusiopathiae* may occasionally

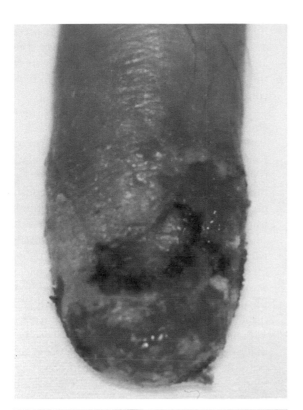

■ FIGURE 10.13

Herpes simplex in AIDS. (Courtesy of F Truchetet, France.)

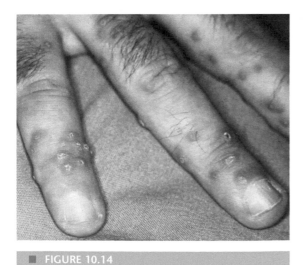

■ FIGURE 10.14

Herpes zoster in AIDS – keratotic lesions. (Courtesy of M Casado, Spain.)

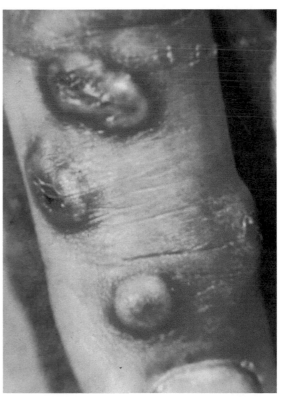

■ FIGURE 10.15

Orf lesions involving the distal digit.

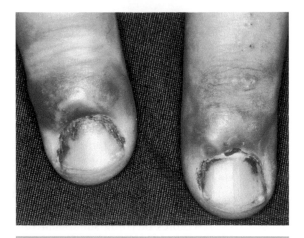

■ FIGURE 10.16

Milker nodule. (Courtesy of RK Scher, USA.)

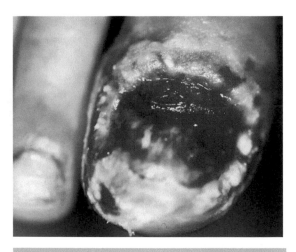

■ FIGURE 10.17

Lectitis purulenta et granulomatosa. (Courtesy of J Bazex.)

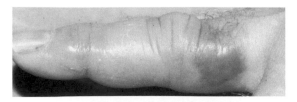

■ FIGURE 10.18

Erysipeloid involving the whole finger. (Courtesy of J Ortiz, Mexico.)

infect a finger tip of a person at risk. It presents as a purplish, painful papule that slowly spreads and exhibits a dusky erythema as it clears from the center. Lymphangitis and paronychia are commonly associated.

Clinically similar is the **'seal finger'** seen in aquarium workers and veterinarians.

Tuberculosis cutis verrucosa (prosector's wart) (Figure 10.19), is an inoculation-type tuberculosis in persons with a good immunity against *Mycobacterium tuberculosis*. It presents as ill-defined nodules with a rough to warty surface, usually on the proximal nail fold.

Atypical mycobacteriosis (Figure 10.20) – particularly swimming pool granuloma due to *Mycobacterium marinum* – can cause violaceous, sometimes more or less verrucous, granulomas of the proximal nail fold that may be slightly tender (probably because of periosteal irritation).[14]

A hard chancre of primary **syphilis** may initially present as a hard infiltrate before it develops into the typical ulcus durum. It may be tender when located under the free margin of the nail.

A case of **leishmaniasis** (Figure 10.21) mimicking erysipeloid has been described, although most leishmaniasis cases around the nail present more usually as a chronic ulcerating paronychia.

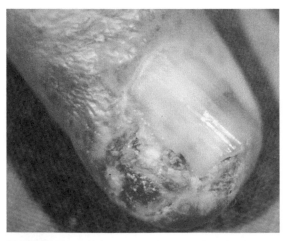

■ FIGURE 10.19

Tuberculosis cutis verrucosa.

Sarcoidosis (Figure 10.22) may involve the distal digit and cause a fusiform swelling of one or more fingers,[15] which is usually painful. The swelling may precede the radiographically visible changes.

Granuloma annulare (Figure 10.23) and **erythema elevatum et diutinum** (Figure 10.24) have also been seen to cause nodules on the proximal nail fold or a markedly thickened proximal nail fold.

Multiple small nodules around the free margin of the proximal nail fold, often with an irregular surface, are characteristic of **multicentric reticulohistiocytosis**, which may or may not be associated with a mutilating arthritis leading to acquired racket nails with shortening of the distal phalanx. Approximately 25% of patients

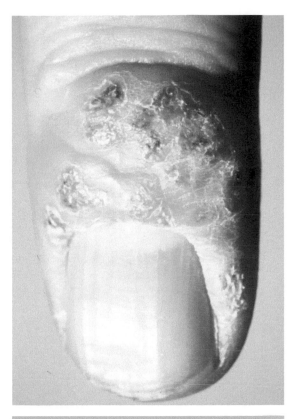

■ **FIGURE 10.20**

Fishtank granuloma.

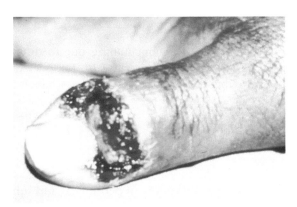

■ **FIGURE 10.21**

Leishmaniasis. (Courtesy of C Arroyo, Colombia. Reproduced from Baran and Dawber's Diseases of the Nails and their Management, 3rd edn. Oxford: Blackwell Science, 2001 with kind permission from Blackwell Science.)

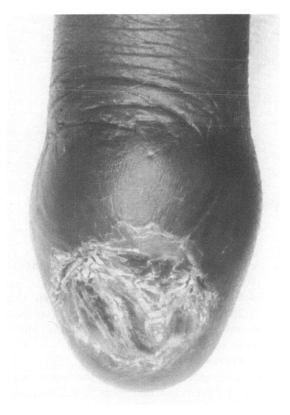

■ **FIGURE 10.22**

Sarcoidosis.

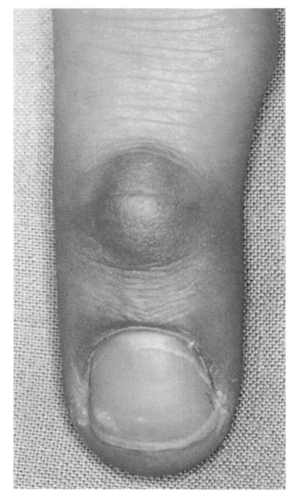

Granuloma annulare. (Courtesy of S Salasche, USA.)

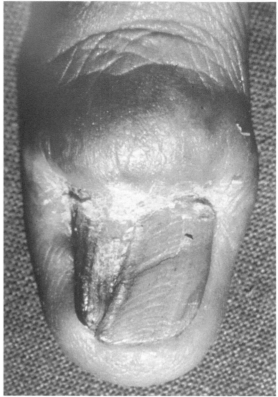

■ **FIGURE 10.24**

Erythema elevatum et diutinum. (Courtesy of G Moulin, France.)

with **multicentric reticulohistiocytosis** (Figure 10.25) have cancer.[16]

Keratosis lichenoides chronica (Figure 10.26) is characterized by linear, lichenoid and warty, keratotic raised papules around the nail, often with an irregular nail surface.[17]

Fibroblastic rheumatism shows nodules over the extensor surfaces of the fingers, including the proximal nail folds. These nodules are firm and flesh-colored.[18]

Blisters around and sometimes even under the nail may mimic a localized swelling or tumor.

Clubbing and pseudoclubbing due to different types of acro-osteolysis may also masquerade as a swelling or tumor of the nail (see Chapter 7).

■■■ PAINLESS TUMORS

■ BENIGN LESIONS

A considerable variety of periungual and subungual lesions may present as swelling or localized tumors. Warts, the most common of these, have already been mentioned.

A **congenital hypertrophic lateral lip** (Figure 10.27) may be mistaken for a tumor of the lateral nail fold in an infant.

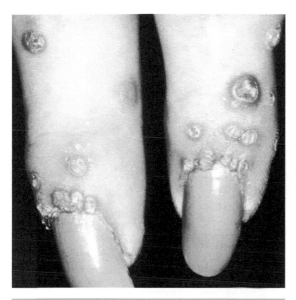

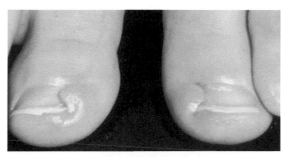

■ FIGURE 10.27

Congenital hypertrophic lateral lip.

■ FIGURE 10.25

Multicentric reticulohistiocytosis papules on the proximal nail fold. (Courtesy of S Salasche, USA.)

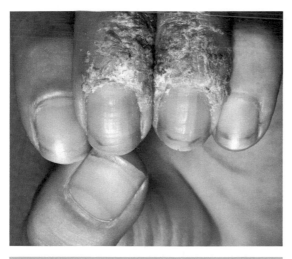

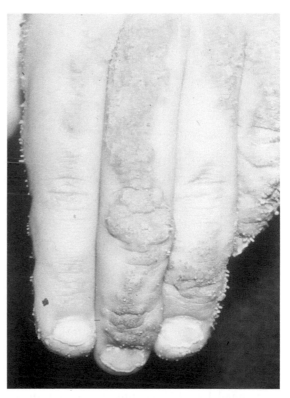

■ FIGURE 10.26

Keratosis lichenoides chronica: warty lesions.

■ FIGURE 10.28

Linear verrucous epidermal nevi.

Linear verrucous epidermal nevi (Figure 10.28) are warty excrescences that usually only affect the perionychial skin, but may sometimes cause a rough surface of the nail plate when they involve the proximal nail fold and its undersurface.

Subungual **papilloma** (Figure 10.29), localized multinucleate distal subungual keratosis,

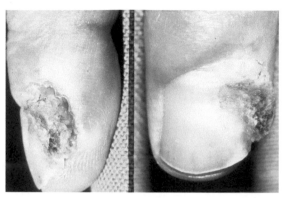

■ FIGURE 10.30
Onycholemmal horn.

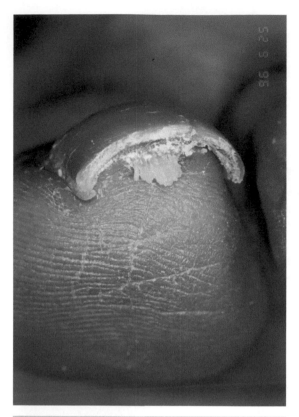

■ FIGURE 10.29
Subungual papilloma.

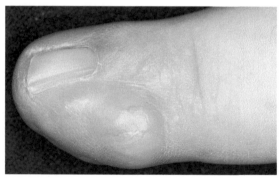

■ FIGURE 10.31
Traumatic cyst. (Courtesy of S Goettmann-Bonvallot, France.)

and onychopapilloma[19] present as small keratotic nodules at the hyponychium under the free margin of the nail plate. They are usually associated with a longitudinal red streak in the nail. Longitudinal erythronychia may be associated with malignancy, especially Bowen's disease.

Subungual **warty dyskeratoma** also causes a small longitudinal rim or a longitudinal red line in the nail.[20,21]

A large wart-like lesion in the lateral nail groove of a finger was identified as an **onycholemmal horn**[22] (Figure 10.30).

Cysts under and next to the nail occur spontaneously or are of traumatic or iatrogenic origin, and may have an epidermal lining (traumatic epidermal cyst), matrical lining (matrix cyst), nail bed lining (onycholemmal cyst), or a mixed lining. Iatrogenic cysts most commonly occur after surgery for an ingrown nail when the lateral matrix horn was not completely removed (Figure 10.31). Traumatic implantation cysts in particular may erode the bone (Figure 10.32) or even grow intraosseously.

Case reports have described a single **subungual syringoma** lifting up the nail plate of a toe and **eccrine syringofibroadenoma** (Figure 10.33) presenting as a keratotic mass replacing the nail or the nail bed.[23]

Eccrine poroma (Figure 10.34) may also occur under or next to the nail. It presents as a pink, slowly growing, singular lesion.[24]

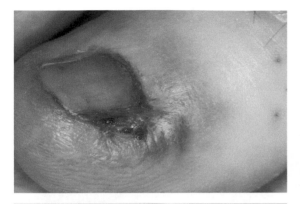

■ FIGURE 10.32

Implantation cyst eroding the bone.

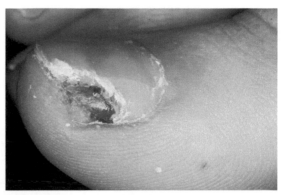

■ FIGURE 10.34

Eccrine poroma. (Courtesy of B Goettmann.)

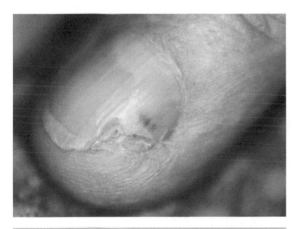

■ FIGURE 10.33

Eccrine syringofibroadenoma. (Courtesy of B Fouilloux, France.)

A **chondroid syringoma** distorted the hallux nail of a 25-year-old woman. An X-ray film revealed lytic bone changes.

Onychomatricoma (Figure 10.35) is a papillomatous tumor of the matrix leading to increased formation of a yellow nail substance with characteristic proximal splinter hemorrhages.[25–27] Depending on its location within the nail, it may give rise to a nodule under the proximal nail fold or assume a paronychia-like feature.

Fibromas occur in different forms, the most frequent of which is acquired digital **fibro-keratoma**. This may be localized on the perionychial tissue and look like a clove of garlic. When it originates from the depth of the proximal nail groove, it forms a sausage-like growth with a keratotic tip that emerges from under the proximal nail fold and lies on the nail plate, causing a longitudinal depression (Figure 10.36). When its origin is in the the middle portion of the matrix, it grows within the nail plate and is covered by a thin lamella of nail plate until this breaks away and shows the tip of the slender fibrokeratoma. Distal from it, the nail plate exhibits a narrow longitudinal depression. In contrast, fibrokeratomas originating from the nail bed cause a rim of the nail plate and may be seen under the nail plate at the hyponychium.

Koenen's tumors (Figure 10.37) are multiple fibromas of the nail apparatus, most commonly originating from the proximal and lateral grooves, but also often from the matrix and the nail bed. Due to their excessive number, they may slowly destroy the nail apparatus. They are round to oval, sometimes hyperkeratotic, nodules that occur in about half of patients with tuberous sclerosis (Bourneville–Pringle disease). Sometimes, they are the only sign of this condition. Nail changes range from longitudinal depressions to malalignment and complete nail overgrowth. When they remain small and multiple, they may resemble onychomatricoma.[28]

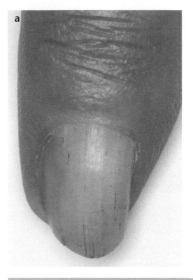
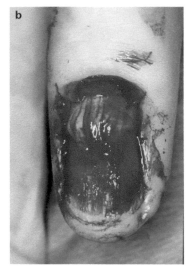
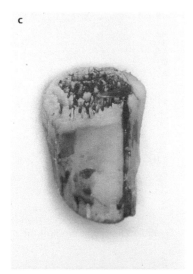

■ FIGURE 10.35

Onychomatricoma: (a) clinical presentation; (b) exposure of the subungual tissue, showing a villus matrical tumor; (c) aspect of the proximal nail plate. (Reproduced with permission from Baran and Kint. Br J Dermatol 1992; 126: 510–5.[25])

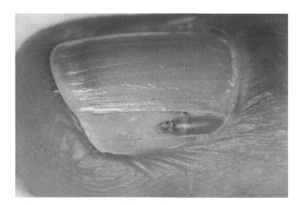

■ FIGURE 10.36

Acquired fibrokeratoma on a narrow longitudinal depression.

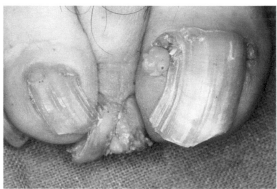

■ FIGURE 10.37

Koenen's tumors interfering with nail growth. (Courtesy of C Beylot, France.)

Matrix fibroma (Figure 10.38) is a rare entity that usually causes a dome-shape flat nodule of the nail matrix and a rim in the nail plate or a deformed, overcurved nail. Its stroma is histologically similar to the fibrous component of onychomatricoma.[29]

About half of **superficial acral fibromyxomas** occur in the nail unit.[30] They are slowly growing lesions that can reach a considerable size and distort the nail, particularly when located in the nail bed (Figure 10.39).

So-called **true fibromas** of the nail are very rare. Depending upon their location within the nail unit, they may present as firm, round to oval, slightly elevated to dome-shaped to polypoid lesions and lift up the nail plate or cause

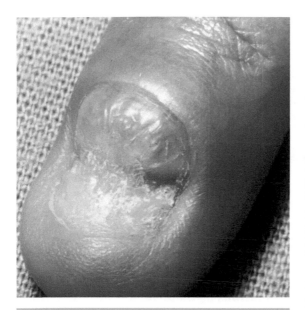

■ FIGURE 10.38

Matrix fibroma. (Courtesy of S Goettmann-Bonvallot, France.)

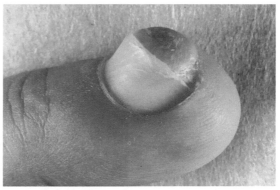

■ FIGURE 10.39

Superficial acral fibromyxoma of the nail bed. (Courtesy of S Goettmann-Bonvallot, France.)

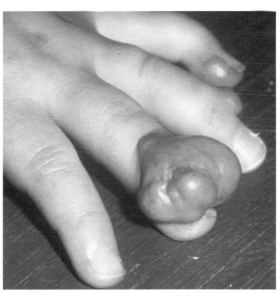

■ FIGURE 10.40

Recurrent infantile digital fibromas.

considerable nail dystrophy.[31] It is not clear whether or not some large fibromas are in fact superficial acral fibromyxomas.

Histiocytomas of the nail apparatus are very rare. We have seen a case of an ungual storiform collagenoma.

Recurrent infantile digital fibromas (infantile digital fibromatosis) (Figure 10.40) are firm to elastic, smooth, round, dome-shaped, reddish nodules, usually on the dorsal or axial surfaces of the the fingers and toes, characteristically sparing the thumbs and big toes. Distortion of the nail may result from large lesions close to the nail. They develop during infancy or may even be present at birth. Occurrence in adolescence or adulthood is exceptional. Often, the fibromas are multiple. They are best left to allow spontaneous resolution, which occurs after the tumoral stage.[32] Histology shows a dense cellular tumor. Approximately 2% of the fibroblasts contain eosinophilic paranuclear inclusion bodies that have no membrane and stain for actin fibers;[32] thus, the tumor is thought to be a myofibroblastoma.

Keloids (Figure 10.41) do not often occur in the nail. We have seen a case with very large keloids of the nail bed and matrix of both big and second toenails after electrosurgery of peri- and subungual warts.

Juvenile hyaline fibromatosis II (Puretić syndrome) (Figure 10.42) is a very rare condition characterized by skin nodules,

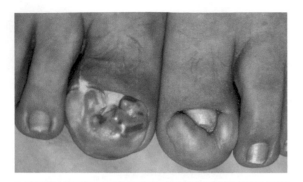

■ FIGURE 10.41

Keloids in epidermolysis bullosa dystrophica. (Courtesy of JC Salas.)

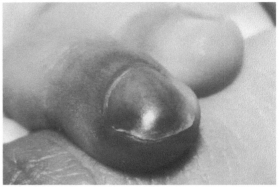

■ FIGURE 10.43

Haemangioma in a 2-month-old child. (Courtesy of O Enjolras, France.)

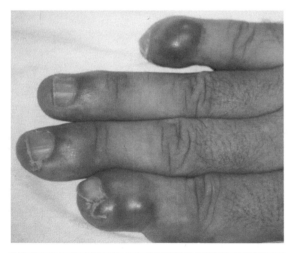

■ FIGURE 10.42

Juvenile hyaline fibromatosis II.

muscle weakness, and flexion contracture of the large joints. It presents with multiple, painless, skin-colored to reddish, hard nodules that have a predilection for the tips of the digits, where they can also cause acro-osteolysis. Histologically, the tumors exhibit a reduction of normal collagen and deposition of a hyaline material that contains 'chondroid' cells. Excision is followed by recurrence.[33]

Vascular tumors are surprisingly rare in the nail apparatus. Infantile **hemangiomas** (Figure 10.43) are very seldom seen. Venous **malfor-** **mations** may arise from bone or soft tissue and lead to diffuse swelling or clubbing.

Arteriovenous malformations (Figure 10.44), both present at birth and acquired, may cause bluish-purple to brown plaques and tumors clinically resembling Kaposi sarcoma. Doppler ultrasound examination usually reveals a shunt.[34]

Angiokeratoma circumscriptum may affect the digits and present with purple to black nodules on their dorsa.

Cirsoid angiomas cause firm subungual nodules that may lead to a red longitudinal streak in the nail or even a split nail. Other lesions that may cause subungual or periungual bluish or reddish tumors are **histiocytoid angioma (pseudopyogenic granuloma)** and **angiolymphoid hyperplasia with eosinophilia**,[35] which has been found to be tender and to cause nail splitting. Small reddish nodules at the tips of the toes of children and described under the term of **acral pseudolymphomatous angiokeratoma of children (APACHE)** (Figure 10.45).

Pyogenic granuloma (Figure 10.46) is the most frequent vascular lesion of the nail apparatus. It is an eruptive angioma that may occur anywhere in the nail, probably after a small penetrating injury. It starts as a small red nodule on

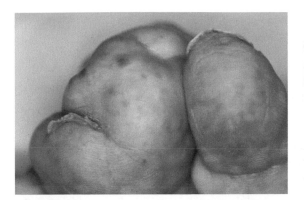

■ FIGURE 10.44
Arteriovenous malformation. (Courtesy of C Lepeytre, France.)

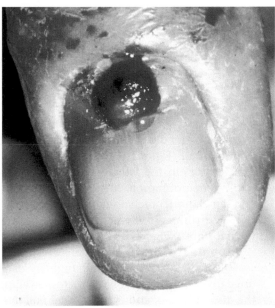

■ FIGURE 10.46
Pyogenic granuloma perforating the base of the nail plate, following trauma.

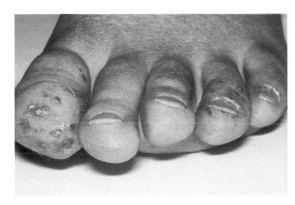

■ FIGURE 10.45
Acral pseudolymphomatous angiokeratoma of children (APACHE) syndrome. (Courtesy of M Dahl, UK.)

the nail fold or at the hyponychium, which soon becomes erosive and develops an epithelial colarette. When located on the proximal nail fold, it may impinge on the matrix and cause a longitudinal depression in the nail plate. Sometimes, it grows through the nail after perforating trauma or prolonged friction (Figure 10.47). Clinically similar lesions of granulation tissue have been seen during treatment with retinoids,[36] cyclosporine, and indinavir.

A characteristic condition, termed **coccal nail fold angiomatosis** (see Figure 5.12), has

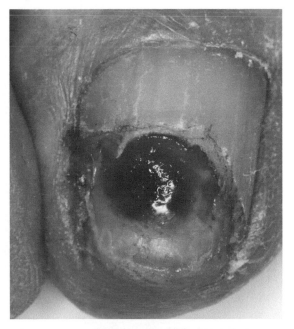

■ FIGURE 10.47
Pyogenic granuloma after frictional microtrauma against the shoe.

been observed in young persons after cast immobilization that presented pyogenic granuloma-like tumors growing out from under the proximal nail fold. It is associated with Reil–Beau lines or even onychomadesis of the affected digits. It may be a particular type of reflex sympathetic dystrophy.

A variety of other conditions may resemble pyogenic granuloma or granulation tissue: ingrown nail (Figure 10.48), benign and malignant tumors in the lateral nail groove and fold (erosive neurofibroma, Merkel cell carcinoma,[37] and (amelanotic) melanoma).

A **lymphangioma** demonstrates a flat subungual tumor (Figure 10.49).

Lipoma is rare in the nail area[38] (Figure 10.50). It may be localized subungually or periungually, leading to clubbing or gross swelling of the distal phalanx and even subtotal nail dystrophy. One case has been reported with a tender and painful swollen distal thumb phalanx.

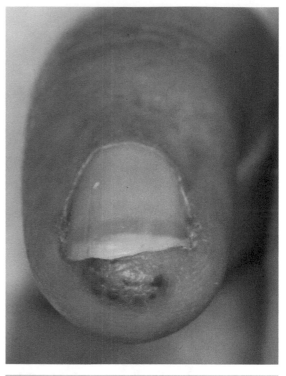

■ FIGURE 10.49

Lymphangioma of the distal digit. (Courtesy of B Richert, Belgium.)

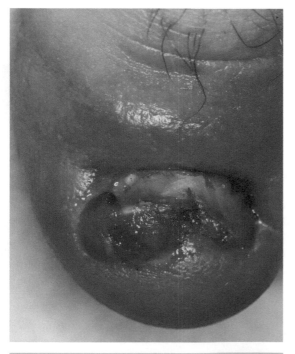

■ FIGURE 10.48

Granulation tissue associated with an ingrown nail.

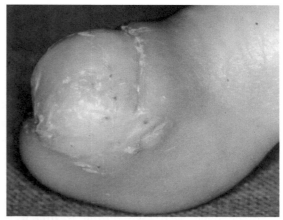

■ FIGURE 10.50

Lipoma involving the nail bed. (Courtesy of A Fanti, Italy.)

Myxomas have been described in subungual localizations and periungually. Depending on their size and site, they may cause clubbing, nail deformity, elevation of the nail from the nail bed, or a circumscribed periungual nodule.[39]

Angiomyxoma may destroy a large portion of the nail (Figure 10.51).

Myxoid pseudocysts (dorsal finger cyst, mucus cyst, distal dorsal ganglion) (Figure 10.52) are degenerative lesions that most frequently occur in the proximal nail fold of elderly persons. Women are more frequently affected than men. Less than 10% occur on the toes. They present as slightly raised to dome-shaped, skin-colored to glassy, firm to fluctuant nodules that cause a longitudinal depression on the nail due to pressure on the matrix. **Heberden nodes** (Figure 10.53) are almost always associ-

ated, and are thought to be of etiological relevance by some authors.[40] They tend to rupture at the undersurface of the proximal nail fold, releasing a gelatinous mucinous material into

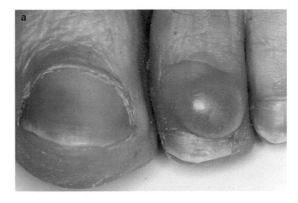

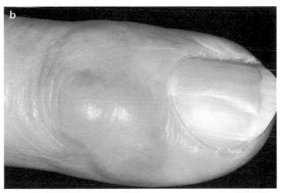

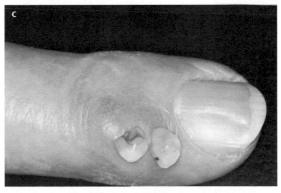

(a) Myxoid pseudocyst of a toenail. (b) Myxoid pseudocyst of a finger. (c) The same patient as in (b), after release of the gelatinous material.

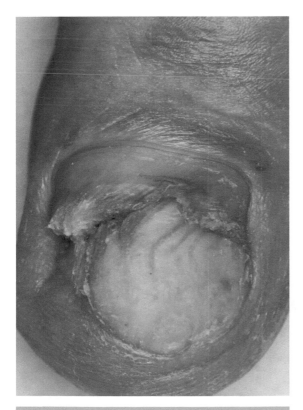

Angiomyxoma of the nail bed.

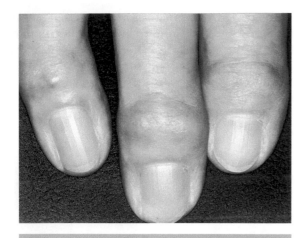

■ **FIGURE 10.53**

Heberden nodes associated with myxoid pseudocyst.

the cul-de-sac. About 30% extend under the matrix (Figure 10.54) and nail bed, but purely subungual myxoid pseudocysts also occur. These cause a swelling over the proximal nail fold, hemitransverse overcurvature, and a characteristic violaceous hue of the proximal nail plate. Transillumination (diaphanoscopy) is positive. There is still a dispute as to whether the lesions are ganglia of the distal interphalangeal joint. However, systematic histopathological examination, including electron microscopy and immunohistochemistry, has failed to reveal any cyst lining. Early lesions always show a circumscribed myxomatous focus with slowly increasing central concentration of mucin until this merges into large mucin lakes and compresses the lateral walls, giving the aspect of a cyst. However, with time, about 80% of the lesions

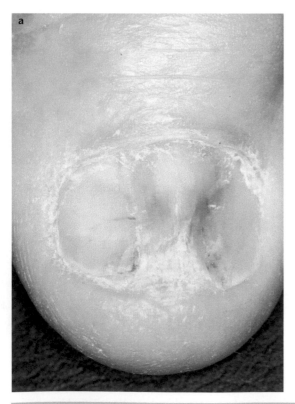
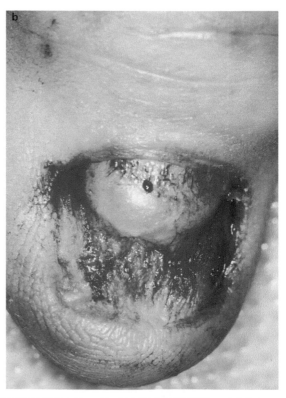

■ **FIGURE 10.54**

(a) Subungual myxoid pseudocyst. (b) The same patient, showing the tumor after nail avulsion.

develop a connecting stalk with the distal interphalangeal joint, which is visualized intraoperatively after intraarticular injection of sterile methylene blue.

Gross papillomatous growths may cover the toenails in excessive cases of **pretibial myxedema**.

Osteoma cutis has presented as firm nail bed tumors.[41]

Subungual calcifications are very frequent and may present as subungual nodules or in the hyponychium (Figure 10.55).

Nodular calcification may be congenital, and presents as a slowly growing, hard, yellowish-white warty nodule at the side of a finger or toenail. Radiographs show a dense mass that consists of multiple calcified fragments adjacent to the distal phalanx.[42]

Neurofibromas (Figure 10.56) are very rare in the nail region. They are apparently of the solitary type, as we have not seen ungual neurofibromas in neurofibromatosis type 1 (von Recklinghausen's disease). They may present as a subungual nodule or mass, resemble an ungual fibroma, distort the entire nail, or cause ridging, clubbing or nail dystrophy.[43]

Thickening of the periungual skin due to systematized **fibrillar neuromas** has been observed.[44] A **Pacinian neuroma** in the distal phalanx was shown to impair finger flexion.[45]

True neuromas of the proximal nail fold presented with marked thickening of the proximal nail fold in a case of multiple mucosal neuroma syndrome.

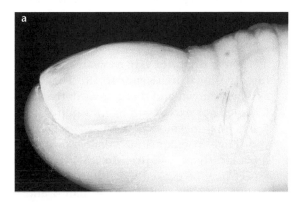

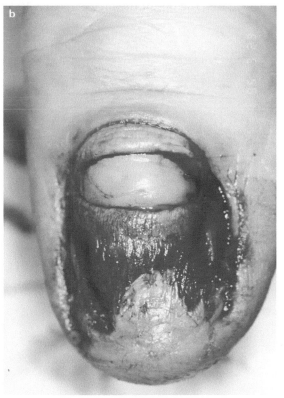

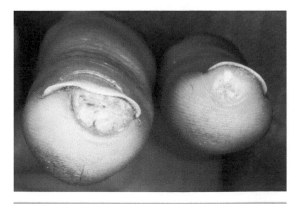

■ FIGURE 10.55

Distal subungual calcification. (Courtesy of C Beylot, France.)

■ FIGURE 10.56

(a) Neurofibroma: clinical presentation. (b) The same patient: exposure of the tumor after nail avulsion and transverse section of the lunula.

Subungual perineurioma may present as a monodactylous clubbing or a red, pea-sized nodule, well demarcated in a distal subungual location[46] (Figure 10.57).

Nerve sheath myxoma should no longer be included under the neurothekeoma rubric.[47]

Soft tissue chondroma has caused swelling and nail distortion.[48]

Papular **melanocytic nevi** are not so rare on the distal phalanx (Figure 10.58). They are usually light brown and dome-shaped; their diameter does not exceed 5 mm in acquired lesions. Congenital melanocytic nevi, however, may be very large, papillomatous, dark brown, and of irregular shape. A **pseudo-Recklinghausen** aspect may be evoked when hundreds of intradermal nevi are found on the hands and feet, including the tips of the digits[49] (Figure 10.59).

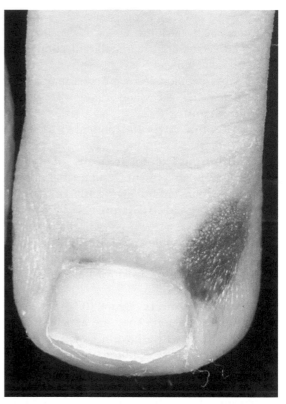

■ **FIGURE 10.58**

Melanocytic nevus.

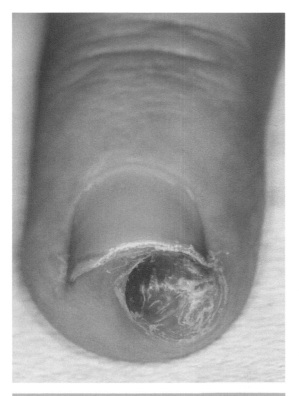

■ **FIGURE 10.57**

Distal subungual perineurioma.

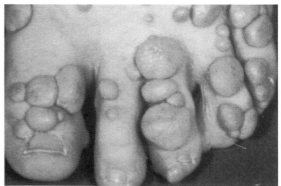

■ **FIGURE 10.59**

Pseudo-Recklinghausen tumors. (Courtesy of C Beylot, France.)

Blue nevi are rare in the distal phalanx[50] (Figure 10.60).

■ MALIGNANT LESIONS

Squamous cell carcinoma is a slowly growing and therefore usually painless tumor that may affect almost every area of the nail apparatus. In situ carcinoma, usually called **Bowen's disease** (Figures 10.61 and 10.62), may present with a plaque-like elevation on the proximal nail fold, which may or may not be covered with a hyperkeratotic scab or an even verrucous hyperkeratosis. It may thus resemble a wart and may occur on more than one digit.[51] Fibrokeratoma-like growths have also been described[52,53] (Figure 10.63). **Invasive squamous cell carcinoma** often develops as a hard, frequently keratotic, nodule. It may ulcerate and mimic pyogenic granuloma.

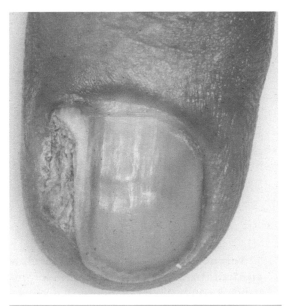

■ **FIGURE 10.61**

Bowen's disease associated with longitudinal melanonychia.

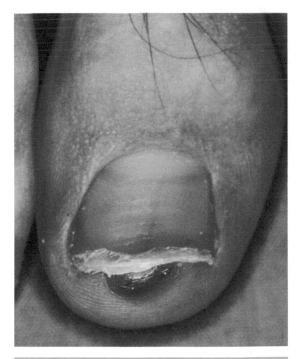

■ **FIGURE 10.60**

Blue nevus. (Courtesy of L Requena, Spain.)

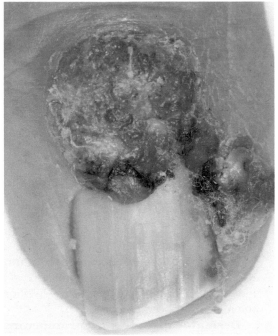

■ **FIGURE 10.62**

Bowen's disease: wart-like lesion.

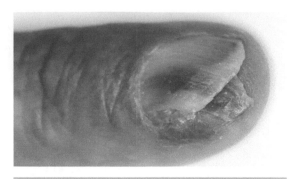

■ FIGURE 10.63

Subungual fibrokeratoma-like Bowen's disease.

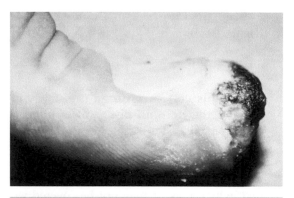

■ FIGURE 10.64

Carcinoma cuniculatum. (Courtesy of BM Coldiron and RC Freeman, USA.)

Verrucous carcinoma and **carcinoma cuniculatum** (Figure 10.64) are low-malignancy squamous cell carcinomas that very rarely occur in the nail apparatus. They tend to give rise to a diffuse swelling of the tip of the digit.[54] Characteristically, a creamy smelly substance can be expressed from the lesion.

A **malignant proliferating onycholemmal cyst** (Figure 10.65) in the thumb of a 74-year-old women was described that destroyed most of the nail and caused considerable bone resorption.[55] Another carcinoma thought to derive from the nail bed has been termed **onycholemmal carcinoma.**[56] This presented with a pyogenic granuloma-like aspect and a slowly enlarging ulcer, eventually causing osteolysis and destroying the nail.

Malignant sweat gland tumors of the nail unit are exceedingly rare. Their clinical appearance is nonspecific and the diagnosis requires histopathological examination. They either present as an ulcerated nodule[57] or as a tender mass.

A single case of a **sebaceous carcinoma** at the radial aspect of the distal phalanx of the index finger causing an increasing swelling of the region has been described.[58]

Dermatofibrosarcoma protuberans is very rare in the distal phalanx[59] (Figure 10.66). It may present as a round, rubbery firm nodule impairing nail growth. One case was painful.

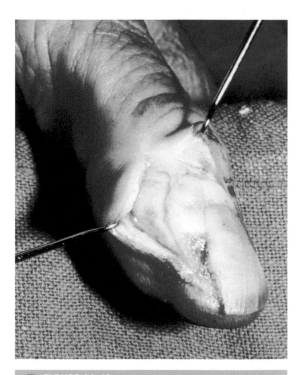

■ FIGURE 10.65

Malignant proliferating onycholemmal cyst. (Courtesy of E Alessi, Italy.)

Kaposi sarcoma (Figure 10.67) often occurs in peripheral locations of the toes. In the classical form, it usually presents as bluish-brown tumors of the feet and toes, slowly overgrowing

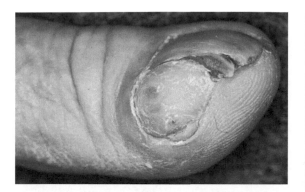

■ FIGURE 10.66

Dermatofibrosarcoma protuberans. (Courtesy of
A Bories, France.)

the nail. AIDS-related Kaposi sarcoma is usually
more generalized, but both subungual and periungual localizations have been described.

Melanomas (Figure 10.68) usually start as
inconspicuous pigmented spots or longitudinal
melanonychia, but one-quarter to one-third are
amelanotic from the beginning. With time, they
grow to sizable nodules that may resemble pyogenic granulomas due to their denuded, oozing
surfaces. In lateral position, melanomas may
look like ingrown nails. Sometimes the tumor is
jet-black, sometimes only partly pigmented or
completely without any visible melanin.
Histopathological examination of any bleeding
mass removed is therefore mandatory.

■■ ■ **PAINFUL TUMORS AND
      SWELLINGS**

■ BENIGN TUMORS

Keratoacanthoma (Figure 10.69) of the tip of
the digit, particularly of the nail, is a rapidly
growing, but benign, painful lesion that usually
appears as a single, painful tumor.[60]

Multiple ungual keratoacanthomas are
very rare[61] (Figure 10.70). The most typical clinical appearance is a subungual keratotic nodule
from which a keratin plug can be expressed.

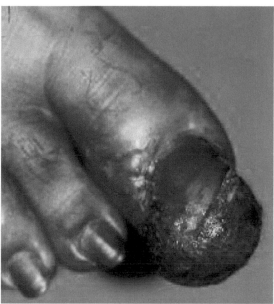

■ FIGURE 10.67

Kaposi sarcoma in an AIDS patient. (Courtesy of
C Aquilina, France.)

Rarely, these may lead to ill-defined swelling of
the entire nail region. Their tendency to spontaneous involution is less pronounced than that of
cutaneous keratoacanthomas, and they tend to
grow rather vertically, compared with the more
horizontal growth of cutaneous lesions. The pain
is probably due to the tendency of the lesion to
erode the bone of the terminal phalanx.
Spontaneous regression with reossification of the
bone defect has been reported.

**Painful keratotic subungual and peri-
ungual keratotic tumors** (Figure 10.71) may
develop in patients with **incontinentia pigmenti**, usually between puberty and the third
decade[62,63] (see also Chapter 9).

Tender keratotic nodules developed on the
tips of the index fingers of a young man who was
addicted to gambling, with an average of 5–7
hours of slot machine use daily for the previous
7 years. The condition was termed **'slot
machine finger'.**[64]

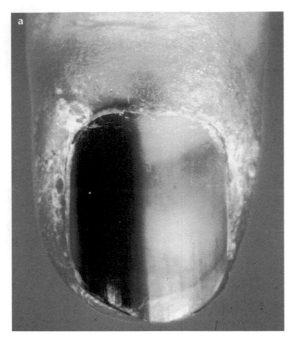

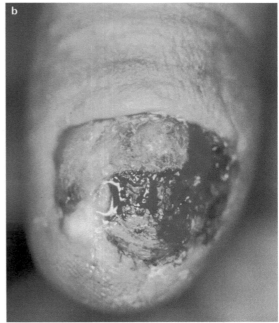

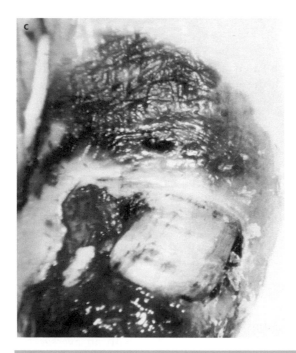

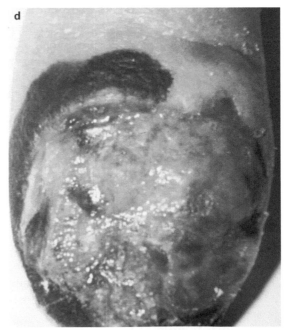

■ FIGURE 10.68

(a) Acromelanoma. (b) Achromic melanoma. (c) Advanced melanoma with partial destruction of the nail and Hutchinson's sign. (d) Advanced melanoma with disappearance of the nail plate and Hutchinson's sign.

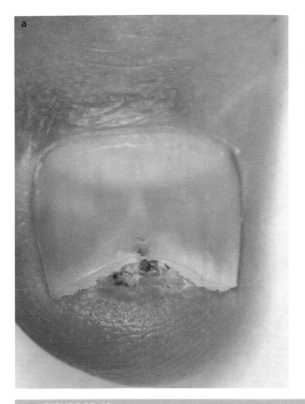
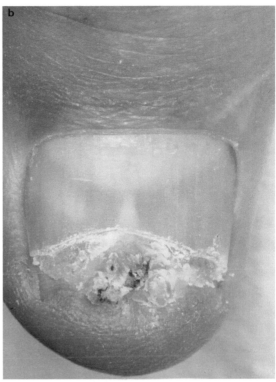

■ FIGURE 10.69

(a) Distal subungual keratoacanthoma. (b) The same patient after nail debridement.

Arteriovenous fistulae (Figure 10.72) are also called **aneurysmal bone cysts** and present as a rapidly growing, painful bulbous enlargement of the distal phalanx of young persons.

Eccrine angiomatous hamartoma in sub- or periungual location has been described twice. It is a reddish-brown painful lesion. It is a characteristic lesion composed of mature eccrine glands in a very vascular stroma.[65,66]

Angioleiomyoma may present as a relatively firm nodule under the nail or emerging from the hyponychium[67] (Figure 10.73).

Glomus tumor is the best known subungual tumour (Figure 10.74) although it is quite a rare lesion.[68] Glomus tumors occur mainly in the hand, specifically in the finger tips and subungually. They are characterized by intense, frequently pulsating, pain that can be provoked or exacerbated by the slightest trauma, such as shock and cold. Placing an ice cube on the nail may trigger pain radiating up to the shoulder. Probing helps to localize the glomus tumor, which is not always exactly where one can see the bluish-red spot shining through the nail (see Chapter 9). Clinically, a violaceous round to oval spot is seen through the nail plate; rarely, a more or less circumscribed swelling can be observed in the immediate surrounding of the nail. A radiograph sometimes exhibits an impression in the underlying bone. High-resolution magnetic resonance imaging allows more precise location of the tumor.

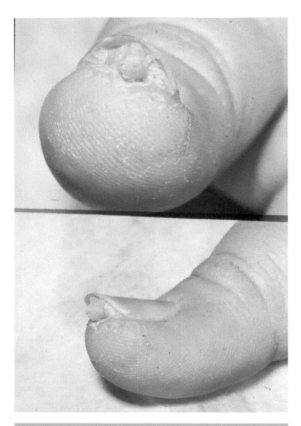

■ FIGURE 10.70

Mutiple nail keratoacanthoma.

Traumatic **neuromas** (Figure 10.75) may occur anywhere in the nail apparatus and give rise to tender nodules on the nail fold or rims in the nail when located in the matrix or nail bed.

Subungual **chondroblastoma** usually presents as a tender to painful, slowly growing enlargement of the affected distal phalanx. A case has been described that started as a nodule, which disappeared spontaneously and developed into a swelling resembling an ingrown nail of the little toe. An X-ray revealed an expansive, partially calcified tumor of the terminal phalanx.[69] Histopathology differentiated it from other more common subungual lesions of osteocartilaginous origin, such as exostoses, osteochondromas, chondromas, and osteoid osteomas.

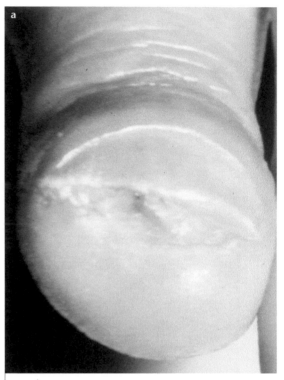

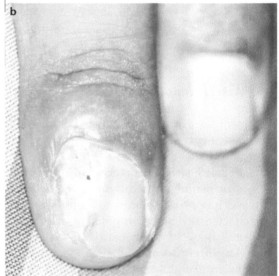

■ FIGURE 10.71

Incontinentia pigmenti: (a) subungual keratotic tumor with distal nail bed involvement; (b) keratotic tumor involving the ventral aspect of the proximal nail fold. (Part (a) courtesy of DS Nurse, Australia.)

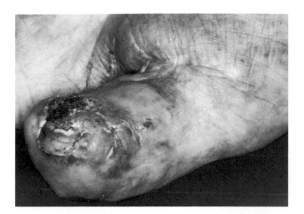

■ FIGURE 10.72

Arteriovenous fistulae. (Courtesy of O Enjolras, France.)

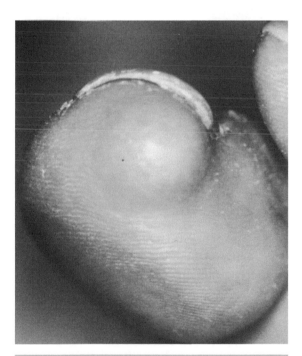

■ FIGURE 10.73

Angioleiomyoma.

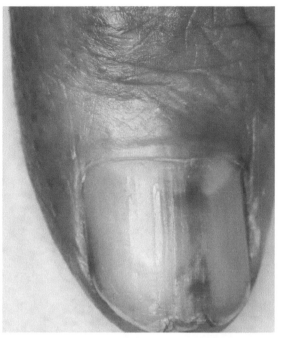

■ FIGURE 10.74

Longitudinal melanonychia associated with glomus tumor.

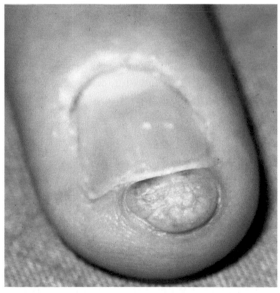

■ FIGURE 10.75

Distal neuroma.

Exostoses (Figure 10.76) occur most commonly on the distal–dorsomedial aspect of the big toe. They are stone-hard tumors, often levering up the nail plate. They are probably due to repeated trauma, as they are frequently seen in

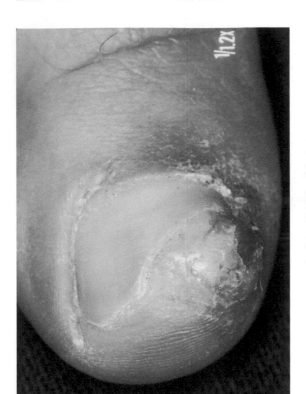

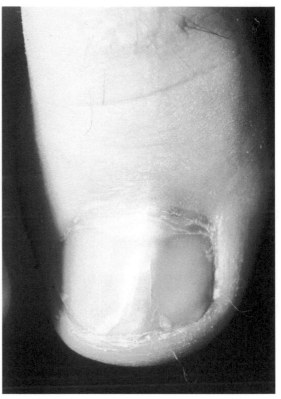

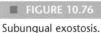

■ **FIGURE 10.76**

Subungual exostosis.

■ **FIGURE 10.77**

Hereditary multiple exostoses syndrome affecting a toenail. (Courtesy of S Goettmann-Bonvallot, France.)

ballet dancers.[70] However, they may be localized anywhere in the nail unit, and cause severe malpositioning or nail dystrophy and even mimic paronychia or an ingrown nail. They are rare in fingers. Bone fragments after fracture of the terminal phalanx may resemble subungual exostosis. Subungual **osteochondromas** are clinically identical to exostoses, with even the histological differences being minimal.

In the **hereditary multiple exostosis syndrome (diaphysal aclasia)** (Figure 10.77), involvement of the terminal phalanx is relatively rare. It may lead to stone-hard tumors, nail malalignment, anonychia, or elevation of the nail plate.[71] When the condition affects the terminal phalanx, it usually involves several digits. It is important to note that there is a risk of

malignant degeneration to chondrosarcoma, except for the distal phalanges.

Enchondroma (Figure 10.78) is the most frequent of all bone tumors of the hand, but is rare in the terminal phalanx. It is a slowly enlarging, painful lesion, which may cause a bulbous enlargement of the distal phalanx, with corresponding nail changes, clubbing, paronychia-like changes, or a subungual tumor lifting the nail plate.[72] It leads to rarefaction of the bone and eventually to pathological fracture. Polyostotic cases are frequent.

Similar nail changes are seen in **enchondromatosis (Ollier's chondrodysplasia)**, often in an extreme form. In **Maffucci syndrome (enchondromatosis with multiple soft tissue hemangiomas)** (Figure 10.79), gross

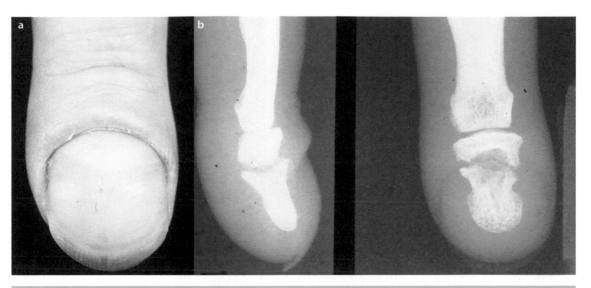

■ **FIGURE 10.78**

(a) Enchondroma of the distal phalanx. (b) X-ray of the same patient. (Courtesy of PD Samman, UK.)

deformation of the distal phalanx with tumors and nail dystrophy occurs.[73]

Osteoid osteoma (Figure 10.80) is a painful lesion causing swelling or clubbing of the distal

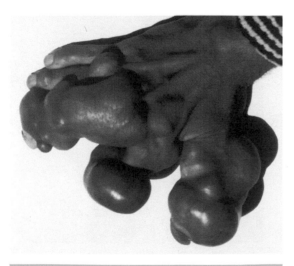

■ **FIGURE 10.79**

Maffuci syndrome. (Courtesy of A Yazidi, Morocco.)

phalanx and a characteristic nagging pain, which is most intense at night. About 8% of all osteoid osteomas occur in the distal phalanx, usually in young persons and twice as frequently in men as in women.[74] Increased sweating has been observed. Radiology shows a circumscribed small area of hyperdensity with a central rarefaction.

Giant cell tumor of the bone is another painful neoplasm that may involve the distal phalanx. It may expand the cortex to two or three times the diameter of the original size, thus causing a bulbous enlargement. Pathological fractures are frequent.

Synovialoma may be localized in the dorsal aspect of the distal phalanx, presenting as relatively hard skin-colored nodules (Figure 10.81), under the nail or in the pulp, causing a bulbous swelling or clubbing.[75]

Oxalate granulomas have been seen in a patient with renal insufficiency and a 20-year history of hemodialysis. They presented as small tender subungual nodules seen under the free margin of the nail.[76]

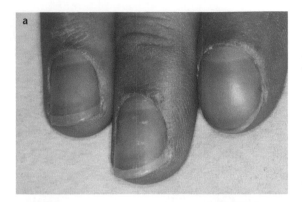

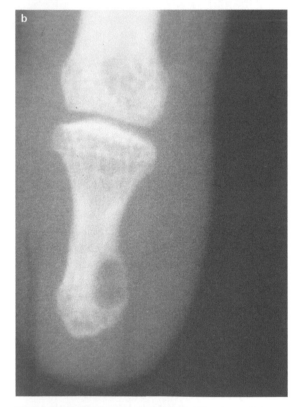

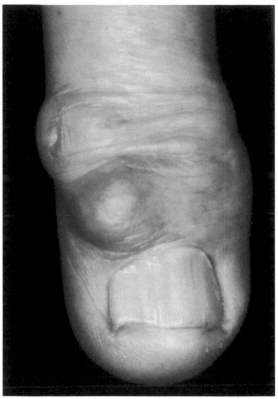

■ **FIGURE 10.81**

Synovialoma (giant cell tumor) involving the proximal nail fold.

■ **FIGURE 10.80**

(a) Osteoid osteoma: pseudoclubbing of the index finger. (b) The same patient: X-ray showing bone sequestration.

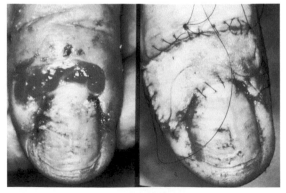

■ **FIGURE 10.82**

Basal cell carcinoma of a finger before and after surgery. (Courtesy of L Goldberg, USA.)

■ MALIGNANT LESIONS

Basal cell carcinoma (Figure 10.82) is very rare in the nail apparatus. It usually presents as a chronic paronychia associated with pain and granulation tissue. Most are located on fingers, with only two having been described on toes.[77]

Sarcomas are exceedingly rare in the nail region. They are insidiously growing, commonly painful lesions. Different types have been described: osteogenic (the differential diagnosis is fibro-osseous tumor of the digits), 'phalangeal', epithelioid, xanthomatous giant cell, epithelioid leimyosarcoma, fibrosarcoma, **chondrosarcoma** (Figure 10.83), haemangiosarcoma, epithelioid angiosarcoma, and Ewing sarcoma. All of these require histopathological examination for diagnosis. Depending on the type and time of diagnosis, a swollen distal phalanx or an oozing mass with loss of the nail may be seen.

Metastases to the nail apparatus and digital tip (Figure 10.84) are rare, with about 160 cases having been reported.[78,79] They are characteristically painful, as most of them primarily affect the bone of the terminal phalanx. The most common clinical appearance is that of clubbing of one or two digits, with a livid to bluish-red color, of a chronic paronychia, or of nail dystrophy. Bronchial carcinoma is the most frequent

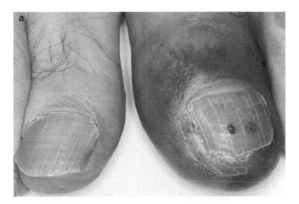

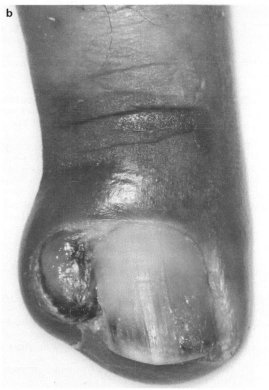

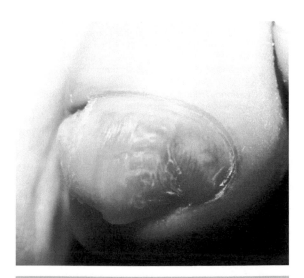

■ FIGURE 10.83

Chondrosarcoma of a distal phalanx of a toe. (Courtesy of S Goettmann-Bonvallot, France.)

■ FIGURE 10.84

(a) Lung metastasis involving the distal phalanx.
(b) Lung metastasis involving the periungual soft tissue of a finger.

primary malignancy (about 50% of cases), but many other carcinomas have been reported, including breast, kidney, colon, rectal, and parotid carcinomas.

■■■ REFERENCES

1. Fournié B, Viraben R, Durroux R, et al. L'onycho-pachydermo-périostite psoriasique du gros orteil. Rev Rheumatol 1989; 56: 579–82.
2. Marghéry MC, Baran R, Pages M, Bazex J. Acropachydermie psoriasique. Ann Dermatol Vénéréol 1991; 118: 373–6.
3. Jury CS, Fleming C, Kemmett D. Severe nail dystrophy associated with painful fingertips. Diagnosis: psoriatic onychopachydermoperiostitis (POPP). Arch Dermatol 2000; 136: 925–30.
4. Narang T, Kanwar AJ. Ectopic nail with polydactyly. J Am Acad Dermatol 2005; 53: 1092–3.
5. de Berker D, Lever LR, Windebank K. Nail features in Langerhans' cell histiocytosis. Br J Dermatol 1994; 130: 523–7.
6. High DA, Luscombe HA, Kauh YC. Leucemia cutis masquerading as chronic paronychia. Int J Dermatol 1985; 24: 595–7.
7. Borrego L, Rodriguez J, Bosch JM, Castro V, Hernandez B. Subungual nodule as manifestation of multiple myeloma. Int J Dermatol 1996; 35: 661–2.
8. Voigtländer V, Hartmann AA, Adam W, Friedrich W. Mycosis fongoïde. Etiologie inattendue d'un eczéma chronique des mains avec gigantisme digital. Ann Dermatol Venereol 1988; 115: 1512–14.
9. Chang P, Baran R, Villaneuva C. Juvenile xanthogranuloma beneath a finger nail. Cutis 1996; 58: 173–4.
10. Kato N, Uehara H, Matsubara M. A case report of EMO syndrome showing localized hyperhidrosis in pretibial myxedema. J Dermatol 1991; 18: 598–604.
11. Fernandez-Diaz ML, Herranz P, de Lucas R et al. Atypical herpes zoster in a patient with AIDS. J Eur Acad Dermatol Venereol 1995; 5: 62–6.
12. Amichai B, Grunwald MH, Abraham A Halevy S. Tense bullous lesions on fingers. Arch Dermatol 1993; 129: 367–9.
13. Eichmann A, Baran R. Lectitis purulenta et granulomatosa. Dermatology 1998; 196: 352–3.
14. Horn MS. *Mycobacterium marinum* infection. J Ass Mil Dermatol 1981; 7(2): 25.
15. Micalizzi C, Parodi A, Rebora A. Nail dystrophy in sarcoidosis. Eur J Dermatol 1997; 7: 509–10.
16. Lesher JL, Allen BS. Multicentric reticulohistiocytosis. J Am Acad Dermatol 1984; 11: 713–23.
17. Panizzon R, Baran R. Keratosis lichenoides chronica. Akt Dermatol 1981; 7: 6–9.
18. Vignon-Pennamen MD, Navran B, Foldes C, et al. Fibroblastic rheumatism. J Am Acad Dermatol 1986; 14: 1086–8.
19. Baran R, Perrin C. Longitudinal erygthronychia with distal subungual keratosis. Onychopapilloma of the nail bed and Bowen's disease. Br J Dermatol 2000; 143: 132–5.
20. Higashi N. Focal acantholytic dyskeratosis. Hifu 1990; 32: 507–10.
21. Baran R, Perrin C. Focal subungual warty dyskeratoma. Dermatology 1997; 195: 278–80.
22. Haneke E. 'Onycholemmal' horn. Dermatologica 1983; 167: 155–8.
23. Fouilloux B, Dutoit M, Cambazard F, Perrin C. Clear cell syringofibroadenoma (of Mascaró) of the nail. Br J Dermatol 2001; 144: 625–7.
24. Goettmann S, Marinho E, Grossin M, Bélaich S. Porome eccrine sous-unguéal. A propos de deux observations. Ann Dermatol Venereol 1995; 122 (Suppl 1): S147–8.
25. Baran R, Kint A. Onychomatrixoma. Filamentous tufted tumour in the matrix of a funnel-shaped nail: a new entity. Br J Dermatol 1992; 126: 510–15.
26. Goettmann S, Drapé JL, Baran R, et al. Onychomatricome: 3 nouveaux cas, intérêt de la résonance magnétique nucléaire. Ann Dermatol Venereol 1994; 121: S145.
27. Haneke E, Fränken J. Onychomatricoma. Dermatol Surg 1995; 21: 984–7.
28. Haneke E. Intraoperative differential diagnosis of onychomatricoma, Koenen's tumours, and hyperplastic Bowen's disease. J Eur Acad Dermatol Venereol 1998; 13 (Suppl 1): S119.
29. Haneke E. The spectrum of ungual fibromas. In: Book of Abstracts, Dermatology 2000, Singapore, 1998.
30. Fetsch JF, Laskin WB, Miettinen M. Superficial acral fibromyxoma: a clinicopathologic and immunohistochemical analysis of 37 cases of a distinctive soft tissue tumor with a predilection for the fingers and toes. Hum Pathol 2001; 32: 704–14.
31. Baran R, Perrin C, Baudet J, Requena L. Clinical and histological patterns of dermatofibromas (true fibromas) of the nail apparatus. Clin Exp Dermatol 1994; 19: 31–5.
32. Duran-McKinster C, Herrera M, Reyes-Mugica M, Ruiz-Maldonado R. Infantile digital fibromatosis: spontaneous regression in three cases. Eur J Dermatol 1993; 3: 192–4.
33. Kan AE, Rogers M. Juvenile hyaline fibromatosis: an expanded clinico-pathologic spectrum. Pediatr Dermatol 1989; 6: 68–75.
34. Kadono T, Kishi A, Onishi Y Ohara K. Acquired digital arteriovenous malformation: a report of six cases. Br J Dermatol 2000; 142: 362–5.
35. Ward KA, Sheehan Al, Kennedy CTC. Angiolymphoid hyperplasia with eosinophilia (ALHE) of the digit. Br J Dermatol 1996; 135 (Suppl 47): 43.
36. Baran R. Retinoids and the nails. J Dermatol Treat 1990; 1: 151–4.
37. Goldenhersh MA, Prus D, Ron N, Rosenmann E. Merkel cell tumor masquerading as granulation tissue on a teenager's toe. Am J Dermatopathol 1992; 14: 560–3.
38. Richert B, André J, Choffray A et al. Periungual lipoma: about three cases. J Am Acad Dermatol 2004; 51: S91–3.
39. Sanusi D. Subungual myxoma. Arch Dermatol 1982; 118: 612–14.
40. Zook EG. Ganglions of the distal interphalangeal joint. In: Krull EA, Zook EG, Baran R, Haneke E. Nail Surgery. A Text and Atlas. Philadelphia: Lippincott Williams & Wilkins, 2001: 209–12.

41. Burgdorf W, Nasemann T. Cutaneous osteomas. A clinical and histopathologic review. Arch Dermatol Res 1977; 260: 121–35.
42. Winer LH. Solitary congenital nodular calcification of the skin. Arch Dermatol Syph 1952: 66: 204–11.
43. Baran R, Haneke E. Subungual myxoid neurofibroma on the thumb. Acta Derma Venereol 2001; 81: 210–11.
44. Altmeyer P, Merkel KH. Multiple systematisierte Neurome der Haut und der Schleimhaut. Hautarzt 1981; 32: 240–4.
45. Altmeyer P. Histologie eines Rankenneuroms mit Vater-Pacini-Lamellenkörper-ähnlichen Strukturen. Hautarzt 1979; 30: 248–52.
46. Baran R, Perrin C. Subungual perineurioma: a peculiar location. Br J Dermatol 2002; 146: 125–8.
47. Fretsch JF, Laskin WB, Miettinen M. Nerve sheath myxoma. Am J Surg Pathol 2005; 29: 1615–24.
48. Dumontier C, Abimelec P, Drapé JL. Soft-tissue chondroma of the nail bed. J Hand Surg 1997; 22B: 474–5.
49. Lycka B, Krywonis N, Hordinsky M. Abnormal nevoblast migration mimicking neurofibromatosis. Arch Dermatol 1991; 127: 1702–4.
50. Soyer HP, Kerl H. Congenital blue naevus with lymph node metastases and Klippel–Trenaunay syndrome. Eur Soc Ped Dermatol Clin Case Rep – Dia-Klinik, 1984: 28–9.
51. Baran R, Gormley D. Polydactylous Bowen's disease of the nail. J Am Acad Dermatol 1987; 17: 201–4.
52. Haneke E. Epidermoid carcinoma (Bowen's disease) of the nail simulating acquired ungual fibrokeratoma. Skin Cancer 1991; 6: 217–21.
53. Baran R, Perrin C. Pseudo-fibrokeratoma of the nail apparatus: a new clue for Bowen disease. Arch Dermatol 1994; 74: 449–50.
54. Coldiron BM, Brown FC, Freeman RC. Epithelioma cuniculatum of the thumb: a case report and literature review. J Dermatol Surg Oncol 1986; 12: 1150–4.
55. Alessi E, Zorzi F, Gianotti R, Parafiori A. Malignant proliferative onycholemmal cyst. J Cut Pathol 1994; 21: 183–8.
56. Alessi E, Coggi A, Gianotti R, Parafiori A, Berti E. Onycholemmal carcinoma. Am J Dermatopathol 2004; 26: 397–402
57. Requena L, Sanchez M, Aguilar P Ambrojo P, Sanchez Yus E. Periungual porocarcinoma. Dermatologica 1990; 180: 177–80.
58. Kasdan ML, Stutts JT, Lassan MA Clanton JN. Sebaceous gland carcinoma of the finger. J Hand Surg 1991; 16A: 870–2.
59. Coles M, Smith M, Rankin EA. An unusual case of dermatofibrosarcoma protuberans. J Hand Surg 1989; 14A: 135–8.
60. Baran R, Goettmann S. Distal digital keratoacanthoma: a report of 12 cases. And review of the literature. Br J Dermatol 1998; 139: 512–15.
61. Haneke E. Multiple subungual keratoacanthomas. Zbl Haut-GeschlKr 1991; 159: 337–8.
62. Abimelec P, Rybojad M, Cambiaghi S, et al. Late, painful, subungual hyperkeratosis in incontinentia pigmenti. Pediatr Dermatol 1995; 12: 340–2.
63. Montes CM, Maize JC, Guerry-Force ML. Incontinentia pigmenti with painful subungual tumors: a two-generation study. J Am Acad Dermatol 2004; 50(Suppl): S45–52.
64. Chaudhry SI, McGibbon D. 'Slot machine' finger: an occupational dermatosis? Clin Exp Dermatol 2005; 30: 90–1.
65. Gabrielsen TO, Elgjo K, Sommerschild H. Eccrine angiomatous hamartoma of the finger leading to amputation. Clin Exp Dermatol 1991; 16: 44–5.
66. Sanmartin O, Botella R, Alegre V, Martinez A, Aliaga A. Congenital eccrine angiomatous hamartoma. Am J Dermatopathol 1992; 14: 161–4.
67. Baran R, Requena L, Drapé JL. Angioleiomyoma mimicking glomus tumour in the nail matrix. Br J Dermatol 2000; 142: 1239–41.
68. Van Geertruyden J, Lorea P, Goldschmidt D, et al. Glomus tumours of the hand. A retrospective study of 51 cases. J Hand Surg 1996; 21B: 257–60.
69. Castanedo-Cazares JP, Lepe V, Moncada B. Subungual chondroblastoma in a 9-year-old girl. Pediatr Dermatol 2004; 21: 452–3.
70. Sebastian G. Subunguale Exostosen der Großzehen, Berufsstigma bei Tänzern. Dermatol Mschr 1977; 163: 998–1000.
71. Baran R, Bureau H. Multiple exostoses syndrome presenting with anonychia on a single finger. J Am Acad Dermatol 1991; 25: 333–5.
72. Wawrosch W, Rassner G. Monströses Enchondrom des Zeigefingerendgliedes mit Nageldeformierung. Hautarzt 1985; 36: 168–9.
73. Tilsley DA, Burden PW. A case of Maffucci's syndrome. Br J Dermatol 1981; 105: 331–6.
74. Foucher G, Lemarechal P, Citron N, Merle M. Osteoid osteoma of the distal phalanx. A report of four cases and review of the literature. J Hand Surg 1987; 12B: 382–6.
75. Richert R, André J. Latero-subungual giant cell tumor of the tendon sheath: an unusual location. J Am Acad Dermatol 1999; 41: 347–8.
76. Sina B, Lutz LL. Cutaneous oxalate granuloma. J Am Acad Dermatol 1990; 22: 316–17.
77. Mikhail GR. Subungual basal cell carcinoma. J Dermatol Surg Oncol 1985: 11: 1222–3.
78. Baran R, Tosti A. Metastatic bronchogenic carcinoma to the terminal phalanx of the toe. Report of 2 cases and review of the literature. J Am Acad Dermatol 1994; 31: 259–63.
79. Cohen PR. Metastatic tumors to the nail unit: subungual metastases. Dermatol Surg 2001; 27: 280–93.

Page numbers in *italics* refer to tables and figures.